What others are sayi
Bedroom:

"Most mates stay too busy or settle for perfunctory sex and miss out on God's sacred adventure of fun, creative lovemaking. The Reids unpack practical Scriptural guidelines that can turn married roommates into lovers: become proactive, learn about your mate, talk about sex, experience the Gospel, set an action plan, and above all— vow to be intentional and follow through! A must read for couples who desire the awesome experience of a creatively intimate sex life."
— Dr. Doug Rosenau, author of *A Celebration of Sex* and co-founder of Sexual Wholeness

"...this book covers what your parents didn't tell you—but should have!"
— Craig Groeschel, Pastor of Lifechurch.tv and author of *The Christian Atheist*

"...fantastic & freeing!"
— Chris & Angie Wheelus, *Center for Relational Growth*

"...Honest, real, insightful, biblical, encouraging, edifying...I wish I'd had this book when I was a new husband."
— Barrie & Eileen Jones, *One Accord Marriage Ministry*, U.K.

"...a courageous book by a courageous couple for such a time as this. We need LTB in the counseling arena."
— Terry Phillips, *GraceLife Family Ministries*

"...much to appreciate."
— Sandra Glahn, co-author, *Sexual Intimacy in Marriage*

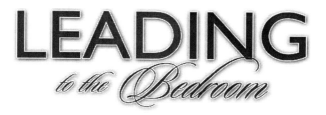

LEADING
to the Bedroom

*The Christian Couple's Path
to Greater Sexual
Intimacy & Freedom*

David & Katie Reid

InnerMan Resources
Carrollton, GA

Leading to the Bedroom
The Christian Couple's Path to
Greater Sexual Intimacy and Freedom
published by InnerMan Resources
InnerManResources.com

© 2010 by David B. Reid

ISBN: 978-0-9827111-1-8

Unless otherwise indicated, Scripture quotations are taken from THE HOLY BIBLE, NEW INTERNATIONAL VERSION®. Copyright © 1973, 1984 by International Bible Society, used by permission of Zondervan Publishing House.

Although the authors have exhaustively researched all sources to ensure the accuracy and completeness of the information contained in this book, we assume no responsibility for errors, inaccuracies, omissions, or any inconsistency herein. Readers should use their own judgment and/or consult a relationship expert for unique applications to their individual situation.

Library of Congress Cataloging-in-Publication Data

Reid, David & Katie.
    Leading to the Bedroom: The Christian Couple's Path to Greater
    Sexual Intimacy and Freedom / by David & Katie Reid.
        230 p. cm.
    Includes bibliographical references and index.
    ISBN: 978-0-9827111-1-8
1. Sex in marriage. 2. Sex—Religious aspects. I. Title
HQ31. R8425   2010

Printed in the United States of America
10 11 12 13 14—10 9 8 7 6 5 4 3 2 1 0

To the Lord Jesus Christ,
Who has given us all things richly to enjoy,
Apart from You, I am nothing.

And for my bride, my beauty,
Katie,
you are the greatest gift I've been given.

And for my Abbie and Ben,
the twin joys of my life,
may you joyfully experience these truths
in the first year of your marriage
instead of the thirteenth.

And to the body at Peachtree Church.
It is my great joy and privilege
to be your undershepherd.
Thank you for your love, support, and encouragement.

Arise,
my darling,
my beautiful one,
and come with me.

—The Greatest Song 2:10

Contents

List of Figures

About the Authors

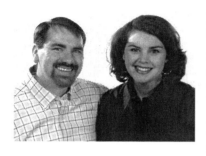 David Reid (Th.M. 2002, Dallas Theological Seminary) is the founding pastor of Peachtree Community Church in Villa Rica, Georgia.

Katie serves as volunteer director of Peachtree's Women's Enrichment Ministry. Married 15 years with two energetic young children and challenging ministries, David & Katie know how busyness can hinder oneness in marriage.

In local church ministry, David & Katie have often taught biblical marriage principles and counseled couples. They have a passion to see couples experience a sweet journey like theirs—to greater oneness and sexual intimacy.

Foreword

A tremendously exciting Movement of sexual growth and revival is mushrooming in the evangelical church. A growing number of God's servants are feeling the Holy Spirit's prompting to unveil His truth about sexuality and create a practical theology of sex that can transform lives and relationships. Thirty years after hearing God's call to help Christians deal with sexuality more effectively, I am humbled to watch the creative Trinity in this 21st Century fashion a Movement—with books, sermons, conferences, academic classes, articles, etc.—that is bringing sexual intimacy, wholeness and healing to the Body of Christ.

David and Katie Reid have joined this rapidly expanding Movement with a powerful new book for enhancing marital sexual intimacy. I can list many reasons this book has a critical message to teach and an important place in helping couples create deeper sexual intimacy. Let me start with my belief that for the church to overcome its sexual inhibitions and lack of practical sexual wisdom—Christian leaders must teach a sexual message grounded in Scripture.

In *Leading to the Bedroom*, David Reid uses his seminary training to develop a practical theology that can indeed help married roommates become lovers again. In a gripping manner, he exegetes well-known Scriptures and brings helpful insights into the meaning of sex and the beauty of marital lovemaking throughout the book. Not only does the reader feel safer with this biblical wisdom, but David also brings a new appreciation for how the Bible can really guide us in our sexuality and marital lovemaking.

I particularly enjoyed the book's development of the idea of "soul sex." For many years, I have taught that our sexuality in general and particularly erotic, romantic lovemaking should be a three-dimensional soul sex involving the physical, psychological and spiritual aspects of our being. So often in our culture, we focus on the body and orgasms rather than see that a crucial part of sexual desire is for intimacy and completion—not climaxes. As so often is stated in present Christian literature, the big "O" is for Oneness and not Orgasm. Soul sex reaches unselfishly into nurturing and fulfilling one another as mates the way the Creator originally intended.

One of my hopes for this book is that the bottom line encouragement for men to become initiators and leaders will not be lost in meaningless debating about complementarian (husbands have headship in marriage) versus egalitarian (husband and wife are equal) interpretations of Scripture. Please suspend your biases and look at the bigger picture that is portrayed in *Leading to the Bedroom*. The Reids are practically trying to effect needed change as they state that men: have greater testosterone and overall a greater sex drive, are more left-brained with a logical focus on the task at hand, crave respect and significance, thrive on taking initiative and pursuing their Eve, and are commissioned to be leaders.

Building on this foundation, this book in a wonderful way says to men: "Quit complaining and grousing about a poor sex life and blaming your wife for having a low desire. Lead! It could be it's not her low sexual desire at all but your lack of leadership and giving her the emotional support she needs to open her body to you in response. You aren't even taking the initiative to create conversations about sex and discussing your desires. Don't gripe and do those common male responses of getting angry or going passive—LEAD."

Compellingly, the Reids' encourage wives: "Pay attention, if you are willing to practice that great Christian virtue submission and trust God's and your husband's leadership—you will reap some amazing rewards. Your husband is trying to unselfishly understand and serve you as never before, pursuing you and your emotional needs. You as Eve have the alluring power to bring out in your man a sexual aliveness only you as his wife can do. Only you can fulfill and help create a sex life that will become nurturing, connecting, and passionate. He can proactively lead you into an awesome sexual intimacy that will be beyond what you might have hoped for and imagined in your daydreaming as a young woman. Open up, respond and be blessed."

As a sex therapist for the past 32 years having heard almost 50,000 hours of stories, I really applaud the four LEAD principles and process. They are steps I have taken countless times and in a variety of ways to help couples make changes in their marriages and sex lives. David and Katie give so many practical ways to avoid common pitfalls and simple pointers for getting started with advice that is practical and real—a manual that is easy to follow.

1) Learn about Your Mate: So many good marriages with decent sex lives never talk about sex—forfeiting a depth and passion they could enjoy. Creating dialogue is a critical place to begin as each mate steps back from their own reality and empathetically learns about the other. The Reids set helpful guidelines for starting the conversations and outline crucial things to discuss as sex is put on the front burner with its expectations, fears, and individual desires/needs.

2) Experience the Gospel: I get so angry I could slap Adam and Eve silly. God gave them the ability to truly be "naked and unashamed" with a passionate intimacy, soul contentment, and amazing connection. All He asked was their obedience, and they blew it for everyone. Since that time, sex has been going downhill. Only with repentance, disputing lies, and God's grace can our love lives be redeemed. Disputing our misbeliefs and acting on truth is another crucial step in leading to what the bedroom was intended to be by its Creator.

3) Set an Action Plan: The critical third step encouraged by the Reids is where both mates take on humility and servanthood and start making changes. By this point, couples have gathered important data and now with an action plan, they can implement and engage. This is always a very critical place in my counseling with couples. Are they willing to let their mate change and take on new attitudes and roles? Will they courageously, with God's help, try new and uncomfortable behaviors? Wow, an action plan can revolutionize a marriage, often in slow, and at times faltering, steps that will in time make such a difference.

4) Do it and Repeat: Thank you, David and Katie, for this final step in the LEAD process. We are all human, and I can guarantee that change will not always be smooth. Action plans will break down. But you start with baby steps, and you then take more baby steps as you step back and work with each couple's unique ways of sabotaging their action plan. Do it—revise—do it—repent again—do it partially—rethink—do it again!

Let me excite you, the reader, with a concluding thought about one of the greatest benefits of working through your marriage to a great sex life. You will understand and experience God with greater feeling, depth and clarity! Why? Because the eternal Trinity created sex as a grand metaphor to reveal Their intimate and creative self. God made man and woman in His very image to be sexual and reflect His joy in intimate communion. Marital lovemaking is the ultimate mysterious portrayal of oneness like Christ and the Bride. How amazing to realize that your creative, intimate love life will bring you constant pictures and insights into the Almighty—helping you become more and more Christ-like.

— Dr. Doug Rosenau, author of *A Celebration of Sex* and co-founder of Sexual Wholeness

Acknowledgements

Great appreciation is due to our dear friends and family who prayed for us and encouraged us in this journey of writing. Too many to name, Katie and I thank God for every word from you that spurred us on. You mean so much to us.

To all our LTB Prayer Team (you know who you are), your prayers and encouragement gave strength to keep going more times than I can count. This project was certainly bathed in prayer. I can't wait to see how He answers for His glory. Thank you and keep praying! This is just the beginning.

A few so encouraged us that this book would not be without them. James & Bryony Hite, your believing in us early on was key to our progress. Chris & Angie Wheelus, you are encouragers par excellence. Without a doubt, you are God's gift to us! David Thornton, your help came at just the right time.

Jason Gupta, your friendship is worth more than you know, and I'm so grateful that God put us next door to each other at Dallas Seminary. When we have our monthly phone call, it feels like you're still across the hall, ready with an encouraging word and a challenging thought. I love it that you don't let me get away with the easy answer but inspire me to struggle through to the right one. I need you in my life.

Kerri Gupta, I don't have the words to show you proper appreciation for the improvements you made with your editing—but I bet you could think of the right ones! You did this while ministering in Ukraine and managing a family. I am so grateful. You are the best!

Doug Rosenau, I am still in awe of God turning your heart to investing in me. You have validated our premise, corrected our flaws, and filled in our gaps. I'm so thankful you have a heart to mentor the next generation. I will listen well!

Most of all, thank you to the Peachtree Church staff and elders who hold my arms up. I love getting to do life with you. And, of course, Katie and I are so grateful to the entire church family that is Peachtree. We are so blessed to shepherd and share life with you. We love you beyond measure and hope to minister God's grace to you with these words!

Finally, Katie, my bride, I thank my God upon every remembrance of you. The Lord blessed me to have the greatest partner in life. You are my best friend, and I can't imagine life without you. As we often say, it's been a full life!

Preface

It was one of those moments that happen too rarely in our hectic lives—when you absolutely know that the God Who created you loves you and you clearly hear His voice. By the grace of God I had been selected, after five years as pastor of the church I planted, for a sabbatical trip to Israel. Not only was the trip a Godsend from the standpoint of experiencing the land where the Bible took place, but this trip also had a particular aim: pastoral rest.

Halfway through this two-week gift of a lifetime, I rose early to watch the sun rise over the Sea of Galilee. Bible, journal, and iPod in hand, I eagerly looked forward to time alone with the Lord.

As I prayed, I began to pour out my heart to my Father, releasing every burden of my first five years of pastoring. I voiced unending concerns and requests, mostly about our church and my keen awareness of my need to grow as a leader. I asked what God had in store for our Body next—you know, ministry stuff. What was the next big thing that I needed to come back and inspire our young congregation to be and to do?

Over the following hour-and-a-half, weights and burdens I didn't realize I was carrying surfaced from deep inside me, and I expressed them all to the One who called me.

Near the end of that time, I found myself in a unique place of emptiness. I had said *everything* that was on my heart. For an extremely rare few minutes in my Twenty-first Century existence, there was complete silence.

In that silence, God began to speak to me. It was as if He said to my spirit: *Now that you're done, there are some things I want to say to you.*

For the next two hours, I began to write what the Lord brought to my mind—mostly gentle (some strong) reminders of things I already knew, certainly all in line with Scripture. Out of six major things I sensed that the Lord was telling me, I was intrigued that only one of them had anything to do with my leadership as a pastor.

The others dealt with my personal life. God pointed to some sin issues that are easy to mask, but are not hidden from Him. He reminded me that He disciplines those sons He loves[1] and that He won't give up on me until He conforms me to the image of His Son.[2]

Also that day, I was re-inspired not to miss a moment of parenting my children. God gave me an intimation that, despite all I dream of doing for Him, perhaps the most important thing my life may ever count for—the most lasting impact I may ever have—is that my children's influence for the cause of Christ might dwarf my own. My greatest legacy, my heart heard, will come from embracing the great responsibility and opportunity of rearing them. All of this was good stuff. It was a great day!

But the one that absolutely floored me, that was not on my radar screen at all—was what God began to tell me that day about my wife's and my sexual intimacy.

~

Now before I tell you what God showed me that day, let me tell you who we are. Katie and I met in the fall of 1993 at a college Christian retreat. It was love at first sight. I pursued her, won her heart, and never had a moment's doubt that she was God's best for me. She says the same.

---

[1] Proverbs 3:12; Hebrews 12:6.
[2] Philippians 1:6; Romans 8:29.

Though it was difficult, we waited and were both virgins on our wedding day, a year and a half later.

Through the providence of God, we waited seven years after marrying to have children. The Lord called me to seminary in the fourth year of our marriage, and Katie whole-heartedly put off her immediate hopes for children to work as a math teacher to put me through school.

Those first seven years without children were wonderful, and—as most couples—we *thought* we were busy. Then came kids, and at the same time we planted a church.

As you might imagine our life now is abundantly full, with a five-year-old and an eight-year-old at the time of this writing and a congregation that is growing and becoming who Jesus redeemed us to be. Full-time ministry has been simultaneously the best and worst thing for our marriage.

Through it all, Katie and I have remained absolute partners; her faith, encouragement, and upbeat attitude are among the greatest blessings of my life.

We've always had a great relationship. In the area of intimacy we've had our highs and lows—just as I suspect you have—which we often chalked up to busyness and pace of life. If I've heard Katie say this once, I've heard it at least twenty-five times: "This is just the summer season of life. It's because we have young children. Things will be better one day."

That's a little of who we are.

~

Now, let's get back to what God told me that day in Israel. Remember, this was out of the blue...I was missing my wife, but issues about our sexual intimacy were not on my mind at all.

The Spirit of God began to say to me: *David, you don't lead your wife in the area of intimacy.*

I considered our sexual intimacy. There were some things that did not please me as much as I would like: certain aspects about our frequency, playfulness, and passion (or lack of these), which did not reflect the ideals we share about what marriage is designed by our Creator to be and what sex in particular is supposed to add to the marriage relationship.

But as I listened that day, God began to pour out surprising ideas to me. I felt compelled to share these insights from the Lord with Katie, so I handwrote sixteen pages for her over the next week. In fact, I honestly don't remember very much about Israel after that point! The rest of the trip I was focused on our relationship and what God was telling me as the head of our family and the leader of our marriage.

I want to share with you the lessons that God taught me as the leader, which I eagerly—and I should add, fearfully—began to communicate to Katie when I returned home.

In the two years since that spring trip, since I began intentionally leading us into intimacy, we have talked more openly and honestly about sex than ever before— and talking isn't the only thing we've done more of, if you know what I mean!

Here are some of the changes in our own intimacy over the last two years (We don't want to boast, but we do want to encourage you that it is worth your time and energy to learn to LEAD.):

- Our average frequency of making love has increased dramatically.
- We've learned to talk about the difficult aspects of marital intimacy—many of them personal issues

which were completely buried yet were holding us back.

- Sex is much more fun than it used to be. I've become more of a romantic and more engaged in courting. Our lovemaking is much more erotic and pleasing to both of us.
- We've experienced a freedom in the area of sex that I only dreamed of two years ago.
- Together we implemented a weekly "fantasy night" where we go beyond "regular" times of sex to intentionally experimenting with ways to keep our intimacy fresh, romantic, and erotic.
- Focusing on our sex life has increased our sense of oneness and strengthened our marriage bond. We feel closer to each other than ever before.

Our enhanced oneness sexually spills over into greater teamwork and warmth toward each other in every area of our life. This is God's design for sex in a marriage relationship. The purpose of *Leading to the Bedroom* is to help you understand why mind, body, and soul oneness is so elusive, and through that understanding, to help you achieve greater oneness in your marriage.

As Katie and I shed the lies of our enemy and I began purposefully LEADing (with great results!), it became clear that the Lord didn't direct me this way in Israel for our marriage alone. Husbands and wives, whether you're newlyweds or well into your journey of marriage, the payoff of learning and applying these truths is huge! Along the way, you'll face some tough challenges, but I believe with all my heart that God can and wants to lead you both to a greater and sweeter soul intimacy, which you can only dream about right now.

Katie's and my desire is to share what God has taught us so that you too can experience greater intimacy and freedom. We are normal people just like you, and our prayer is that this book will encourage you to embark on this satisfying journey back to all that God intended sex to be for married couples.

May you be challenged to LEAD well so you can love passionately!

For His Glory and by His Grace,

David & Katie Reid

Chapter One
Paradise Lost
How the Thief Broke in
and What He Took

Now the serpent was more crafty than any beast of the field...
—Genesis 3:1

The thief comes only to steal and kill and destroy...
—John 10:10

Satan does everything he can to get a couple into bed before they're married and everything he can to keep them out after.
—Author Unknown

Sex would never be the same.

He thought back to their wedding day, the first time he saw her hair touching her bare shoulder, that one-of-a-kind face and figure he had come to love at first sight. She wore a wreath of fresh flowers in her hair, and the pleasant fragrance hinted there were more good things to come.

Though he was not generally the artsy type, his first look at her body inspired him to poetry.

They kissed—slowly and tenderly at first, but then more passionately. Even now, he remembered, her red, full lips tasted like strawberries.

Holding her at arms' length, he couldn't take his eyes off her firm, young breasts—like ripe fruit on a tree. His mind raced at the possibilities—and along with it, his pulse. Her eyes invited him, and, he was soon to discover, the new round fruit seemed perfectly designed to fit into his hands. Instinctively, he caressed and tasted. She let out a surprised sigh, then moaned softly in delight, letting him know it was good for her as it was for him. *Don't stop*, she had said—and he didn't.

He gently explored further down; every part of her body was a feast for his senses. To touch the curve of her hips, to feel her legs wrapped around him, her hands in his—Paradise!

The unique organs below their waists quickly found what they had been made for—realizing that one part fit perfectly into the other was a thrill beyond any he had ever known. He felt simultaneously powerful and vulnerable, as she gave herself fully to him and he to her. The joining of parts began a chain reaction of sensation and symphony of movement together with her that was singularly pleasurable in all his experience.

To be one with his bride was the most joy and pleasure he had ever felt.

To be one with his bride was without a doubt the most joy and pleasure he had ever felt.

But it will never be the same now, he lamented.

She, too, was mourning the loss of oneness and warmth that had marked their relationship from the beginning, but now seemed hopelessly shattered by recent events.

For her, sex took a while longer to get into for sure. But that only seemed to heighten the mutual cooperation and caring of the whole experience.

The intimate conversation and playful innuendo he'd interject throughout the day was a not-so-subtle sign that he wanted her again. Her heart skipped a beat when he would grasp her hand and purposefully interlace fingers so as to have as much skin-to-skin contact as possible. He would serve her in unselfish and delightful ways, frequently giving her an enormous bouquet of colorful and fragrant flowers he'd picked himself. She knew he worked hard to let her know what was on his mind, and all the attention made her feel beautiful and generous. When he whispered in her ear, "I reeeaaally love you!" she knew he meant it.

She smiled for a moment at how good they'd gotten at foreplay. She'd had to teach him to slow down, but she had to admit he'd put his whole heart into studying her desires and responses. She enjoyed his affection and tenderness, and she blessed him with the visual show that he obviously loved. The discovery that almost every part of their bodies had a sensual aspect made them both eager to experiment because the potential for new sexual pleasures seemed endless.

Beyond the physical pleasure, for her, it was the sense of sharing something with him and only him—that's what made their intimacy marvelous. Though she was the more eloquent of the two by far, even she could not quite express the closeness sex brought, but perhaps that was what was greatest about it: when they came together, there was a soul connection much deeper than mere words could create or sustain.

When they came together, there was a soul connection much deeper than mere words could create or sustain.

When they lay naked together, his arms wrapped snugly around her body, she felt secure, warm, one with him, and thankful to God. This was the way life was meant to be.

But all of that seems so far away now, she sobbed to herself.

Adam and Eve sat in silence, markedly distant from one other, still stunned by the magnitude of the consequences of the first sin.

To have reached for something more when they had everything God had so richly provided for them, now seemed, as it was, the most horrible thing in the world. Wanting more had gotten them less—infinitely less. The first couple, mourning in fig leaves, ashamed and alone, thought simultaneously, *This is not the way it was meant to be.*

Handle with Care

Almost ten years of personal pastoral care have taught me that marriages are like fine china: beautiful and priceless in their intended state and use, but fragile and easily broken if not handled with proper care. And precious dishes are breaking all around us, even among those who know Christ.

Some shatter with loud crashes from intentional abuse like a dish thrown against the wall. Others crumble from simple careless neglect, with chips and cracks from day after day of improper wear and tear.

In these cases, often the marriage partners themselves aren't aware of the structural weakening they are introducing by their inattention to the care of their union. Either way, it is a fact observable all around us: marriages can break, and the broken pieces devastate everyone involved.

Marriage, one of God's best-designed blessings for His glory and our good, is suffering the Satanic effects of the Fall.

We have long cited a rising or high divorce rate as a measure of the crisis state of marriage. However, divorce is just the final, most tragic step. Beyond the marriages that actually shatter in divorce, there are thousands more holy unions struggling in varying degrees of distress and brokenness.

Money difficulties or incompatibility are often cited as causes of the fracture, but these are really just symptoms.

At the root of marriage difficulties is a problem as old as the Fall: a loss of oneness. God designed the one-flesh relationship as a protective wall around marriage, with husband and wife safe and secure in a loving, protected, unashamed, unselfish, joy-giving relationship.

> *The root of marriage difficulties is a problem as old as the Fall: a loss of oneness.*

But in the Fall, Satan broke through that protective wall, attempting to steal the oneness God created for Adam and Eve. In its place, he erected a divisive wall between the first couple, tragically evidenced in Adam's defense to God, "That woman you gave me—she gave me the fruit, and I ate it."[3] For the first time in history, husband and wife were not on the same team—man did not see his wife as the mutual helper God created each of them to be. Unfortunately, it would not be the last time.

Figure 1. Before and After the Fall

| Husband Wife | Husband | Wife |

Protective Wall   **Divisive Wall**

God's Intention in Creation

This is not the way it was meant to be. In Genesis 2:7-17, God handcrafted His highest creation. Then He actually breathed His life into him, and placed him in charge of the earth, a paradise God had just created for His glory and Adam's enjoyment. He gave him authority and freedom and one clear rule to demonstrate that he trusted God. God made man to represent Him over all His creation and to receive His love. It doesn't get much better than that...well, actually it does!

After God proclaimed six times that all He had made "was good," one thing in His creation didn't meet His

---

[3] Genesis 3:12 (my paraphrase).

standard. Genesis 2:18 tells us God's opinion of Adam's bachelor status:

18 The LORD God said, "It is not good for the man to be alone. I will make a helper suitable for him."

What follows is an amazing, beautiful, and grace-filled story as God leads Adam to recognize his own incompleteness—and then spectacularly provides for his need. Let's follow along:

*19 Now the LORD God had formed out of the ground all the beasts of the field and all the birds of the air. He brought them to the man to see what he would name them; and whatever the man called each living creature, that was its name. 20 So the man **gave names to all the livestock, the birds of the air and all the beasts of the field.***

In the Old Testament, naming something implies having authority over it. God gave Adam authority over all His creation.

*But for Adam **no suitable helper** was found.*

Can't you see Adam? Aardvark, Female Aardvark...Beaver, Lady Beaver...Camel, Girl Camel... There's definitely a pattern, but there's no one for him. The Hebrew word translated "suitable helper" is *ezer*, which means "one who assists and serves another with what is needed."[4] *Ezer* is not a condescending title. This special companion is much more than a faithful dog who

[4] James Swanson: *Dictionary of Biblical Languages With Semantic Domains: Hebrew (Old Testament)*. electronic ed. Oak Harbor : Logos Research Systems, Inc., 1997, S. DBLH 6468, #2.

fetches your paper. (Whoever said "a dog is a man's best friend" was either single or had missed what marriage is supposed to be!) Many times in the Psalms, the psalmist calls God his *ezer*,[5] and in Hosea 13:9, God calls himself Israel's *ezer*.

But God planned a human helper for Adam also. He arranged this parade of animals and naming exercise specifically to make Adam aware of his need for one to be with him to help him through life. None of them were physically, mentally, emotionally or spiritually like Adam. The parade exaggerated their inappropriateness and foreshadows that Eve, God's gift, is the best fit for Adam.

21 So the LORD God caused the man to fall into a deep sleep; and while he was sleeping, he took one of the man's ribs and closed up the place with flesh.

Today, singles chase after "the one" or fret because there is no one on the horizon to chase. Consider the biblical pattern: Adam rested (he was asleep) while God prepared whom he was to marry. God knows what we need—and how He needs to prepare us before we're married, so we need to rest in the knowledge that "in all things God works for the good of those who love Him, who have been called according to His purpose."[6]

Eve was taken from Adam's *side*, Matthew Henry said, not from his head to rule over him, not from his feet to be trampled on, but from his side to be equal with him, under his arm to be protected, near his heart to be beloved.[7]

---

[5] Psalm 33:20, 70:5, et al.

[6] Romans 8:28.

[7] Matthew Henry, *Matthew Henry's Commentary on the Whole Bible: Complete and Unabridged in One Volume* (Peabody: Hendrickson Publishers, 1991), S. Genesis 2:21.

*22 Then the LORD God **made** a woman from the rib he had taken out of the man, and **He brought her to the man.***

Eve was the missing part of Adam. Husband and wife are literally one flesh, built by God for each other and incomplete until God brings them together. Here is the first wedding with God (her Father) giving the bride away.

23 The man said,
"This is now bone of my bones
and flesh of my flesh;
she shall be called 'woman,'
*for **she was taken out of man.**"*

Adam was overjoyed at his gift from God—that she was like him. Adam called her *ishshah*, "woman," meaning "from *ish* (man)." Essentially, Adam was calling her "Mine."[8] I often ask my wife when I'm overcome with her beauty or love toward me, "Are you really mine?" Adam said with great satisfaction, "You're mine!"

*24 **For this reason** a man will **leave** his father and mother and **be united** to his wife, and they **will become one flesh**.*

Because God ordained one woman for one man from the beginning, the foundation of all marriage is creating a new family unit: leaving your family of origin and establishing a new family with loyalty to and oneness with your spouse. Your relationship is to be so close that God calls it "one flesh." Adam's rib was reunited with his body as husband and wife came together.

---

[8] Matt Chandler. "Sex." Sermon, The Village Church, Denton, TX, May 15, 2005.

*25 The man and his wife were **both naked**, and
they felt no shame.*

God says this is how He created marriage to be. They
were both naked. This means that there were no barriers
between them; they were completely vulnerable with each
other. And it goes without saying that it strongly hints at
sexual oneness. In their intimacy, "they felt no shame"—
there was no reason to be ashamed because this is what
God intended for them.

God said it was not good for man to be alone. His
answer was to create an *ezer*, a beautiful Hebrew word
that means a helping companion. This is a mutual
complementary calling on each marriage partner to assist
each other in whatever ways a spouse will need in life.
God created Eve specifically for Adam, one woman for
one man, gave her to him, and Scripture says, "they were
naked and not ashamed." They were free to know each
other and be fully known. Naked, in paradise with a
partner made just for you, no shame...thank God He's so
good!

A Terrorist Plot

Unfortunately it didn't last long. How did God's
incredible plan for mankind, which included one man and
one woman joined together in oneness, go so terribly
wrong? Genesis 3 tells us it began with a thief. In order to
understand how the enemy steals what God intended for
your marriage, let's consider his first assault:

*1 Now the serpent was more crafty than any of the
wild animals the Lord God had made.*

Later in the progress of God's revelation, we find out that Satan was behind the animated serpent, hiding his identity from the first couple he came to rob.

He said to the woman, "Did God really say, 'You must not eat from any tree in the garden'?"

The Devil's first and consistent word throughout history has been to tempt us to doubt that we can trust the God who made us. After mixing enough of the truth for Eve to let her guard down, he convinced her that God had been withholding something good from her, the chance to be like Him.[9] This struck a chord because she wanted to be more like God. What she failed to realize was that she was already like Him—created in His image. Often the enemy's deception is such: by his trickery, we forfeit contentment when we already have what God has given us to enjoy.

In this first instance of a husband abdicating leadership and going passive, Adam and Eve both ate the forbidden fruit. But afterward, instead of feeling more like God, they experienced a new emotion: shame.

7 Then the eyes of both of them were opened, and they realized they were naked; so they sewed fig leaves together and made coverings for themselves.

The passage doesn't tell us which parts of their bodies they hid. Logic would indicate that it was their mouth and hands—the members they sinned with. But history bears out (up to today) that it was their genitalia, the parts that were different from each other.

One theory supposes that they shone with the glory of God in their created state. When sin separated them from

---

[9] Genesis 3:4.

God, they lost the Divine glow, and this was the reason for their shame.[10]

What is certain is that in addition to severing their relationship with God, the Fall also damaged their relationship with each other. Satan had stolen the *ezer*, helping companionship, God had given them. "Naked and not ashamed" vulnerability had been murdered. "One flesh" closeness was destroyed. The fig leaves hid them from each other as much as from God, for they covered the parts with which they consummated their oneness.

The enemy devastated the protective wall created around their relationship. The divisive wall he craftily replaced it with is evident in Adam's response to God's question about their disobedience:

12 The man said, "The woman you put here with me—she gave me some fruit from the tree, and I ate it."

That marital oneness is a casualty of the Fall is pronounced in God's curse on his sinful Creation. In verse 16b, God says,

"Your desire will be for your husband,
and he will rule over you."

The consequences of sin would be a tragic breakdown of the helping partnership God intended. Respected Hebrew scholar Allen Ross links the woman's "desire" here to the same word in Genesis 4:7—sin's desire to master Cain.[11] In other words, Eve (and her daughters) will tend to continue to kick against the created order of the husband's headship. Men, on the other hand, will tend

---

[10] John Phillips, *Exploring Genesis: An Expository Commentary* (Grand Rapids, MI: Kregel Publications, 2001), 59.
[11] Allen Ross, *Creation & Blessing: A Guide to the Study and Exposition of Genesis* (Grand Rapids, MI: Baker Books, 1987), 146.

to exercise their authority harshly (see the second half of 16b).

The battle of the sexes began that day. In this verse, some see the beginning of godly headship, but they're missing the point. God had already created things the way they were supposed to be. Here, He's declaring that the rebellion they've started against Him will continue as rebellion in their relationship. This is a statement of the curse—it shows how fallen couples will treat each other, not how they should.

> *21 The Lord God made garments of skin for Adam and his wife and clothed them.*
> *22 And the Lord God said, "The man has now become like one of us, knowing good and evil. He must not be allowed to reach out his hand and take also from the tree of life and eat, and live forever."*
> *23 So the Lord God banished him from the Garden of Eden to work the ground from which he had been taken.*
> *24 After he drove the man out, he placed on the east side of the Garden of Eden cherubim and a flaming sword flashing back and forth to guard the way to the tree of life.*

What a tragic end to such a beautiful beginning. That day in the garden Satan declared war on God's created order. He had already rebelled against God Himself in Heaven, and God had put the rebellion down by casting him out of Heaven.[12] Unable to successfully attack God directly, he did what every cowardly terrorist does—he went after His loved ones.

---

[12] Isaiah 14:12-15 (the King of Babylon's arrogance and fall is symbolically indicative of Satan); Luke 10:18.

He set his sights on God's image bearers, His highest
and most treasured creation—and he attacked them with
deadly skill. And in doing so, he rocked the world. He
turned God's created order upside down. God had set up
an ordered hierarchy, with Himself at the top. Man was
God's representative on the earth, with a submissive
helper beside him. Together, humans were given
dominion over the animal world. Satan reversed the order
with an animal (the serpent) deceiving the woman, who
influenced her husband, who disobeyed God. Man and
wife, who were created to always be on the same team,
were now divided.

Figure 2.
God's Created Order Turned Upside Down in the Fall

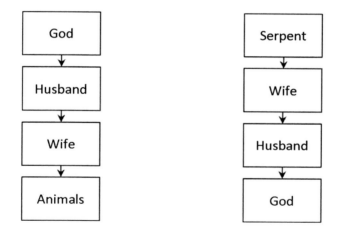

Furthermore, in the Fall, something was broken—
correction, *everything* was broken. When man stopped
trusting God, his relationship with God was shattered.
Not only that, his relationship with the opposite sex was
broken. Sexual intimacy, designed by God to be the most
powerful catalyst to marital oneness, was broken. All
because an enemy came into Eden.

Later, Jesus would tell his followers Satan's true nature. In John 10:10, Jesus said,

"The thief comes only to steal and kill and destroy."

His one purpose, the Lord said, like a thief's, is to take what people have—what belongs to them. That day in the Garden, the Devil put on a snakeskin disguise. He came into the garden with his enticing words, with just enough truth, enough seemingly legitimate justification, and he stole what God had provided.

Among all the catastrophic tragedy of the Fall that day, the enemy tried to steal God's gift of oneness in marriage. He tried to kill intimacy, God's precious gift of knowing and being fully known by someone who was made for you, and you for them. He tried to destroy sex in all its beauty as the great catalyst to greater oneness in marriage.

And from every generation since Adam and Eve, Satan has tried to rob spirit, soul, mind, and body marital intimacy.

A Slough of Schemes

Today, our enemy is systematically and strategically destroying God's design for sexuality just as he was that day in the Garden. There is an ongoing spiritual battle with marriages on the line every day. Fortunately, Katie and I started our marriage with a sense of the spiritual war going on. And, as church planters for eight years, we've had front row seats to the battle in the lives of our congregation. Don't doubt that you and your spouse have a personal enemy with his sights trained on your marriage. Here are some of his favorite tactics:

Lies. He has new lies for every generation. In the Victorian era, the world (influenced by the father of lies) viewed sex as a necessary evil for procreation. Christian women were taught they should not enjoy it—only endure it when necessary. Consequently, prostitution flourished.[13]

In stark contrast, Satan's scheme in the 1960s in America was the "sexual revolution" promising free sex and no rules. Medical statistics can track the explosion of STDs during that time, but the emotional wounds and lingering cultural effects are unfathomable. When sex became unlinked from marriage on a societal scale, the breakdown of the nuclear family followed as evidenced by the proliferation of divorce in the past forty years. Both these historical Satanic plots led humanity further from God's great design for oneness in marriage.

Childhood Experiences. Today, the assault is even greater. The attack begins earlier and earlier in our lives and advances on every side. Girls are made to feel insecure about body image from a pre-teen age. Boys without dads learn about sex (divorced from any teaching about marital commitment) from other teen-aged boys or the hidden magazine that every man seems to have found in his boyhood. I know who put it there—our enemy.

Sexual Abuse. Worse, sexual abuse touches one in four girls and one in six boys,[14] creating a lifetime of wounds and shame (even though it was *not* their fault). These are carried into marriage if not skillfully and tenderly dealt with. My pastoral experience teaches me that most are not.

---

[13] Trevor Fisher, *Prostitution and the Victorians* (New York: St. Martin's Press, 1997), 60.

[14] *ACE Study - Prevalence - Adverse Childhood Experiences,* http://www.cdc.gov/nccdphp/ace/prevalence.htm.

Loss of Purity. The idea that purity is possible has been stolen, by and large, from an entire society, and with it, the precious gift of presenting one's body saved wholly for one's spouse. The wounds from premarital sex are emotional and lifelong. Previous experiences have a way of bringing insecurity and unwanted memories into the marriage bed.

Pornography. The pandemic of pornography in our world is staggering. More money was spent on porn in 2007 than on professional baseball, basketball and football combined—more than $60 billion worldwide.[15]

Because God designed sex to bond us to our spouse, there are chemical things happening in the brain as men look at porn. Porn is addictive, artificial intimacy, driving a divisive wedge between couples like nothing else. The internet has privatized porn (embarrassment about buying it is no longer a barrier), made it live-action, and provided instant access to every home with a computer. Porn sites even advertise through innocuous searches to hook the young and uninitiated.

You don't have to spend much time with men to realize that Satan starts early springing pornography on curious boys who have no idea of the dangerous trap he has set. And many men wrestle with the addiction the rest of their lives, grieving their wives along the way. Satan has staged a coup with pornography.

The allure of pornography is a deception. If the married sex relationship were what God designed it to be, who would want to watch 2D sex? The enemy has so thoroughly deceived husbands and wives about God's gift that is available to them in each other.

---

[15] Mark Driscoll. "The Peasant Princess: Let Him Kiss Me." Sermon, Mars Hill Church, Seattle, WA, September 21, 2008.

Adultery. Physical infidelity, or even just lustful thoughts toward anyone outside the marriage, destroys the beautiful "one flesh" oneness God intended. Entire families are devastated when a spouse falls into this sin.

Worldly Culture. Media and movies have become ever louder and more emotionally powerful voices to shape society's view of what sex should be.[16] The "romantic comedy" genre of film, with young girls and dating couples as its primary target audience, often includes a great-looking infatuated couple sleeping together as a plot twist without the real-life consequences. This is the enemy's "frog in the kettle" strategy to desensitize a whole generation to the sanctity of sexual intimacy. It's working.

The Attack Continues

All of these are ways the enemy steals from us, and there are many others. (It could quickly get overwhelming, no?) In fact, it is nearly impossible to enter marriage unscathed by one or more of these enemy attacks. But if you have the character, maturity, and commitment to pick up a book on marriage, then the enemy is probably waging a more subtle attack on your relationship.

His crafty strategy for you is the same one that has been operating in husbands and wives since the Fall. If your intimate life is a disaster, I can guarantee the enemy has stolen this aspect of your relationship. But even if you'd call it a 9+ on a scale of 1 to 10, I'd wager that what keeps it from being ideal is a lack of true soul-sexual intimacy.

This is the area of marriage Satan has been most intentional, and successful, at stealing. It's been said, wisely, that the Devil does everything he can to get

---

[16] Meanwhile, the church has been almost silent.

couples into bed before they're married, and everything he can to keep them out after.[17]

Remember, before the Fall, there was a perfect protective wall around the relationship between the first man and first woman. Adam recognized this unique relationship when he acknowledged that Eve was "flesh of my flesh"[18]—she was to be part of him like no other created thing (including animals, his own family of origin, and other women). God ordained that "the two shall become one flesh,"[19] designating unselfish teamwork—oneness—as the core value of marriage. His perfect plan placed them in paradise, where "they were both naked and were not ashamed"[20]—no divisive wall between them. Perfect vulnerability, perfect interdependence—the key to each partner's joy lay in the selfless sharing of all of oneself with the other.

Satan's goal was—and is—to tear down the protective wall around a couple's relationship and build up a divisive wall between you, exactly the opposite of God's plan for His creation.

And so he focuses his attack on sex—trying in every way to twist its original design, because sex in marriage is meant by God to be a catalyst for oneness. It is the greatest gift in all creation for couples to draw closer together and to strengthen their marriages. Yet, because of the enemy's success, there is a sex famine among married couples. In almost ten years of pastoral care, I have met an alarming number of married women who report that they can take or leave sex and often would prefer not to have that expectation placed on them. The enemy has effectively stolen God's greatest catalyst to oneness in marriage.

---

[17] Author unknown. Some wise preacher, I suspect.
[18] Genesis 2:23.
[19] Genesis 2:24.
[20] Genesis 2:25.

The Error of Grandpa Adam

In order to understand how he steals soul sex from couples, we've got to look closer at *how* the Fall occurred. It would be convenient to let the story end with Satan's attack—to suggest that all our marital problems, including a lack of oneness, come from Satan and that we are merely helpless victims. But we have a responsibility on our shoulders.

Ever since Adam, husbands have been called to lead their wives. Before Eve was even created, God gave the command to Adam not to eat from the tree of knowledge[21]—it's clear that it was Adam's responsibility to lead his wife to obey God.

But when Satan (who was the most crafty creature in the Garden) came to tempt, he went after Eve. And Adam was silent and followed his wife, instead of leading her to obey God. Adam went passive, and the rest, as they say, is history. Genesis 3 teaches us that a husband who does not lead to God leads to sin. And, in fact, he is one dangerous step away from tragic loss of joy and oneness.

> *Genesis 3 teaches us that a husband who does not lead to God leads to sin.*

Adam's error was going passive when he should have been taking responsibility. I've talked to enough men (and had enough experience myself) to see the fallen pattern play out over and over. We commit Adam's error! It happens in other areas also,[22] but because sex is God's greatest catalyst for oneness, Adam's error is particularly devastating in the realm of intimacy.

There are actually two wrong ways a man can choose to go when he is not experiencing satisfying marital intimacy with his wife. First, he can get angry. Truer words were never written than James 1:20: "Man's anger

---

[21] Genesis 2:16-17.

[22] It may be helpful to consider Adam's error in other areas of your life also.

does not bring about the righteous life that God desires."[23] Angry men build up a divisive wall between themselves and their spouses, moving further away from oneness.

Much more common is Adam's error: going passive. Suppose a wife has a wound the enemy inflicted somewhere along her life. It causes her to shy away from "naked and unashamed" oneness with her husband.

In an attempt to be a loving husband, he suppresses his God-given desire in order (he thinks) to lovingly, sacrificially meet her needs. Also, when she rejects him, shame kicks in, and he finds it embarrassing to ask again. This can lead to a cycle of passivity in the area of intimacy.

He could swallow his pride and help his wife heal her wound and healthily come into the *incredible* world of intimacy intended by God "who richly provides everything for our enjoyment."[24] But, thinking he is being a loving husband, he inadvertently lets her keep her wound instead. They both miss out on the blessing soul sex was meant to be and are more susceptible to the temptation to meet their God-given needs out of the bounds of marriage. Thus, Satan steals from both of them what God provided by giving them to each other.

This cycle of passivity leads to the lowest common denominator (LCD) of sexual intimacy, in which a married couple settles for whatever level of intimacy the most inhibited spouse is comfortable with. The LCD is frustrating to both spouses—even the more inhibited one was designed to enjoy more frequency, fun, freedom, fervor, and feelings—and it restricts "naked and unashamed" sex, the greatest catalyst for oneness that God designed. God meant for us to pursue and enjoy the

---

[23] James 1:20.
[24] 1 Timothy 6:17.

greatest level of intimacy possible—not the lowest common denominator.[25]

Figure 3. Adam's Error – The Passivity Cycle

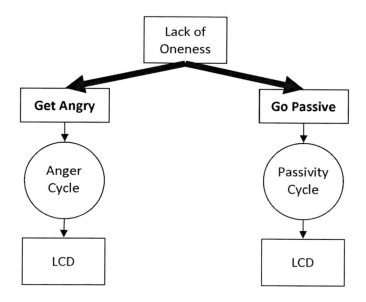

Of all the ways the enemy tries to steal from, kill, and destroy us, he has a specialty for married couples— robbing the soul-sexual intimacy God intended by enemy-inflicted wounds that go unhelped and unhealed through Adam's error of passivity.

Why is that his specialty for couples? Sex is absolutely exclusive in marriage. No one else can please your husband or wife in physical intimacy. That's why Satan loves to steal this gift—that's why He loves to trick couples into taking the LCD route. It puts you in a catch-22 of either missing out on one of the greatest gifts God gave His creatures to enjoy or meeting God-given sexual desires out of bounds.

---

[25] We'll talk more about the LCD in Chapter Three.

One Husband's Revelation

God impressed on me that I was not leading in the area of intimacy as I lead in finances, child-rearing, ministry, and other life decisions in our marriage.

In each of these other arenas, I discern God's will from Scripture and leading of the Holy Spirit and take the lead, even correcting my bride's thoughts and actions if they are not in line with the direction I am receiving as the spiritual head of household.

But not so in our sex life. Because this is a much more "intimate" realm—harder to talk about and tangled with potential issues of shyness, shame, abuse, etc., I had not clearly led in this area as in others. I realized that I had often *thought* I was doing the loving thing and actually heeding "Husbands, love your wives just as Christ loved the church," by being intimate only when she wanted to (and not asking/demanding that my desires be met).

But He showed me that I am called to lead us in sexual intimacy just as surely as He gives me the responsibility to keep the family on track financially.

That's when it dawned on me that we'd been robbed and that my lack of leadership was the same error as Adam's, who abdicated headship when the thief came to steal paradise from his family.

There is Hope

But couples can experience tremendous progress in sexual understanding and freedom as husbands commit to lead in this area and as wives affirm the desire to follow to greater levels of intimacy.

Your growth in intimacy and marriage is a key part of God's ongoing sanctification process to conform you to the image of Christ.[26] Husband, the most incredible gift you can give your wife is to learn to lovingly and selflessly lead as God intended; and wife, learning to respect and follow such a leader is one of the best gifts you can give him. Having experienced the difference between the lowest common denominator and moving toward soul-sexual intimacy, we don't want anyone to settle for less.

Where We're Going

Just by the fact that you started and are still reading this book, you are choosing that you want your marriage to be more than it is now.

What if I could teach you a process that would bless both husband and wife—that would sweeten your soul oneness and spice up your sex life more than you ever thought possible? Wouldn't it be worth it?

John 10:10 says the thief comes to steal, kill, and destroy. And he has. But the good news is that Jesus said, "I have come that they may have life, and have it to the full."[27] He came to redeem and restore what the thief took. He came to give us life back, and the fullest life we can imagine.

Together, we're going to avoid Adam's error and foil Satan's schemes. We're going to exposit key Scriptures on God's intent for sexual intimacy—soul sex, I like to call it. Then, I'll teach you how to LEAD—a process to move to greater oneness, including more passionate intimacy.

Men, God is calling you to lovingly take initiative in your sexual intimacy in order to bless both you and your wife with greater oneness. While you have suppressed your desires and felt frustrated or guilty for asking, your wife has also not been able to be free. She was created to enjoy her sexuality just as you were.

---

[26] Nothing is more Christ-like than to become a selfless giver in your marriage.
[27] John 10:10b.

Wives, you have stunning beauty in your husband's eyes (inner and outer). God made you to respond to your husband's pursuit—to be sassy, flirtatious, to playfully use your charms to heighten your desire for each other. And that kind of joy-giving relationship is closer than you think.

Husbands and wives both have a responsibility—and much to gain. Trust me, this is truth worth applying in your lives. So, take the next step: decide right now that you won't settle for less than what God originally gave (and what Jesus wants to redeem for you). That includes God-blessed sexual intimacy leading to greater oneness. Make a commitment not to settle for the lowest common denominator in your marriage, but to pursue the greatest possible level of intimacy.

Come into the Light

A few years ago, I inherited an old jon boat. It wasn't seaworthy, but I thought it might be a fun project to fix as a hobby. I lugged it to the corner of my yard, where it covered up a boat-sized patch of grass. As a dad and pastor, my spare time didn't come as quickly as I'd hoped. Weeds grew up around the boat, and the lack of light nearly killed all the grass underneath it.

Seasons later, when I did remove the boat, it had become so much a part of the landscape that I had to rip it away from the weeds, which had a stranglehold on it. I had to mow the grass to see the tragic state of my lawn underneath. The boat had left a scar: its perfect image highlighted in bare dirt.

But by the next summer, I was amazed! With just some sunlight, the grass sprang back to life—now I can't even locate the exact spot where my turf was tortured. The healing sunlight revived what was lying dormant.

That's what I believe God wants to do in your sex life. That day in Eden, the enemy threw a blanket over sexual intimacy. He tried to stop the light from coming in. He tried to steal what God provided for husband and wife. And for many of you, it has worked. You lost paradise.

But Jesus went to the Cross so that we might experience a full life (including God-blessed sex in marriage).[28] In order to experience it, we've got to let the light shine into the areas Satan's tried to shroud in darkness. God is inviting you to bring your sex life and God-given desires into the light.[29] That's the invitation of *Leading to the Bedroom*. Take a step into the light. God intended so much more for you.

A Wife's Take

I am completely on board with what Dave is saying—and that is no small statement! It is one thing for a shy girl (me) to choose to be led in intimacy in ways I hadn't before—quite another to decide my husband and I should write about it for anyone to read.

But we both feel a very certain sense of calling about this—that God wants to use what He taught us to encourage oneness in marriages throughout His Kingdom. This has the same feel to it as every clear calling we've experienced...a little fear, the excitement of adventure, a sense of inadequacy, the need for dependence on God, and a feeling of not wanting to miss how He wants to use us.

Look for "A Wife's Take" throughout the book to get a woman's view on things—sometimes we don't see things the same way as our husbands, you know. May the Lord bless you as you lead and follow to greater oneness!

---

[28] John 10:10b.
[29] Ephesians 5:8-14; 1 Peter 2:9.

Chapter Two
Soul Sex
A Theology of Intimacy

How beautiful is your love, my sister, my bride!
How much better is your love than wine...
—Song of Solomon 4:10

Eat, O friends, and drink; drink your fill, O lovers.
—Song of Solomon 5:1b

What you believe about God is the most important thing about you.
—A. W. Tozer

Love Letter

There's a grand dessert offered to us. But we've left it on the tray. Maybe we thought it might be too rich for us. Now, of course, we have enough of the sweet that we can't quite put our finger on what's missing. Some days we get a taste of great dessert, and we love it! Still we fool ourselves that this kind of dessert is for anniversaries, birthdays...special days—not any day.

One of us was tricked by the enemy into thinking that kind of dessert is for "once-in-a-while," and the other one decided not to risk offense by expecting that kind of dessert more often. So, day after day, we do the hard and wonderful work of preparing great meals to sustain us:

we communicate,
we forgive,
we manage money together,
we're raising great kids,
we even serve shoulder-to-shoulder in ministry—

we sacrificially put each other first in a thousand ways for the good and nourishment of our family...

But the enemy has stolen the dessert that God meant for us to enjoy with regular meals. We're missing that the dessert makes the whole meal better. And, honey, the dessert is great!

I want to enjoy dessert with you more frequently, more freely, and more passionately—so badly I can taste it. This is not a selfish ambition; I want you to enjoy our dessert. We were created to...together.

Jesus said He came so our life could be full—scream-my-name-out-loud, come-get-back-in-bed, take-me-in-the-shower, come-home-from-work-now-I've-got-new-lingerie, let's-curl-up-by-the-fire-and-make-love *full* life as Christian husband and wife. When we miss the sweetest part of our meal—the icing on the cake, it's because the enemy has stolen it from us. I will fight for us to get it back.

On cold nights, our family enjoys having a fire in the fireplace. My wife is kind of a purist, so we have a firebox with real wood—none of those convenient gas logs in our home. And we light it the natural way, too—no gas igniter or turning on a light switch. That would be too easy.

As much as I'd like to be that guy who strikes a match to a single sheet of newsprint under some split kindling perfectly arranged to *start* the fire, unfortunately, it's not a skill I possess. I have to have a catalyst—something to jumpstart the reaction. Give me two firestarters, those fuel-drenched modern wonders that light easily and burn long and hot enough to get the wood burning—and we'll have a roaring fire in no time.

God included a kind of firestarter in His plan to ignite true soul intimacy between husband and wife. Think about it. God knew the Fall was coming. Marriage would be difficult at times. Take two completely different people. Bring them together after their formative years, once they're set in their ways, you might say. Each is coming into marriage with different backgrounds, values, and opinions, along with a deep struggle with selfishness—the sinful flesh nature that has plagued God's prized creation since the Fall. Without warmth, passion for each other, and a lifelong commitment to oneness, they'd never make it.

So, God created something that would deepen this all-important bond beyond mere friendship, logic, convenience, or contractual arrangement. Not to mention that in its intended state, this "something" would bring extreme joy and pleasure to both husband and wife.

At the risk of oversimplifying, sex is a firestarter. In fact, sex is the greatest catalyst for marital oneness that God has created. It's hard to get the fire in marriage roaring without it. And it's really hard to stop a fire ignited by this catalyst if started at the wrong time or with the wrong person.

Sex is the greatest catalyst for oneness God has created.

If your marriage is not blazing as it should be, providing warmth for you and your spouse, then it's worth taking a closer look at sex. What all did God mean for it to do in your marriage?

A Theology of Intimacy

For some of you, putting "sex" and "God" together in the same sentence feels sacrilegious. It shouldn't! Sex was God's idea—and He pronounced it "very good."[30]

You may be thinking, with all the important issues in the world, why does God care about the sex life of a Christian man and his wife? Because it is the most powerful unifying act between husband and wife.

---

[30] God's pronouncement of "very good" (Genesis 1:31) came only after Eve, Adam's counterpart, was created.

With so much awkward silence on the topic, along with lies by the enemy, what we need is a theology of intimacy. A. W. Tozer said, "the most important thing about you is what you think about God—because that determines

Sex is the most powerful unifying act between husband and wife.

everything else about you." If you rightly view God as the loving, all-powerful, all-wise Heavenly Father that He is, then it should be easy to view sex in marriage in its proper context as a "good and perfect gift...from above, coming down from the Father of lights."[31] The most important thing about you *is* what you think about God—because that determines how you think about everything else, including sex.

God created this marvelous built-in outlet to make couples closer, contented, and joyful—even to keep you from sinning. Like a fire in your home, in its proper place (the fireplace), it brings warmth and joy. But if it spreads outside its intended context, it can quickly destroy the whole house—even the neighborhood. Sex is just that powerful. We must make sure we know God's design for intimacy if we are to use it to its full potential for good and avoid the devastating misuse of His wonderful gift to us.

If your sex life is not the blazing, warmth-providing blessing God intended, it is very likely connected to a false or deficient view of what He meant it to be.[32] For that reason, we need to understand God's perspective on marital intimacy—so we can think properly about it. So get ready for the sex talk that, odds are, you've probably never heard—from a godly, spiritual perspective.

First, let's define a few terms we'll be using often. These aren't really technical definitions, but more a description of what we mean by them.

---

[31] James 1:17.
[32] Barring any physical issues.

Marriage. Marriage is a covenant relationship instituted by God between one man and one woman. It's the foundational social unit of God's plan for humanity because it is designed for the propagation of society (having children)[33] and the continuing knowledge of God among future generations (spiritual training in the home).[34]

Marriage was created to be a helping relationship.[35] Norm Wright's definition is helpful: "Marriage is an unconditional commitment to an imperfect person for the development of his or her God-given potential."[36] Viewed this way, marriage is to be the pinnacle of unselfishness. You get married for the betterment of your partner, not yourself. You are meant to strive for your partner's best, and ultimately that provides what is best for both of you.

Marriage is the ultimate tool for discipleship. Nobody has as much influence over you as your spouse. God wants to use your marriage to conform you both to the image of Christ. I *love* Gary Thomas' take on marriage: "What if God designed marriage to make us holy more than to make us happy?"[37]

Finally, marriage is a gift for great joy. When God said, "It is not good for the man to be alone," He was declaring His intent to *bless* man with a wife, and vice versa. Companionship, joy, meaning, and, yes, great pleasure are God's design for each partner when He brings two people together in marriage.

Intimacy. Intimacy means closeness. God's highest goal for your marriage is "oneness," a bond closer than any other human relationship. What does intimacy

---

[33] Genesis 1:28.

[34] Deuteronomy 6:1-9.

[35] Genesis 2:18.

[36] Norman Wright, *The Premarital Counseling Handbook* (Chicago: Moody Press, 1992), 15. Wright's definition is slightly altered here to emphasize God's plan for each spouse as the goal as opposed to a selfish self-actualization.

[37] Gary Thomas, *Sacred Marriage* (Grand Rapids, MI: Zondervan, 2000), 5.

according to God's design look like? A few biblical words
are helpful.

Hebrew Words for Intimacy

Pastor Matt Chandler deftly outlines the godly
progression of a relationship using the Hebrew biblical
words for different levels of intimacy. Notice that
intimacy increases as a couple moves toward marriage.
First, there is *ra'ah*, or companionship. This is a deep
level of friendship based on a vulnerable knowledge of the
other person: "You know everything about me—even the
bad stuff, and still you choose to walk with me." You are
blessed if you have a *ra'ah* companion. It is rare in our
world. *Ra'ah* is wonderful, but there is something deeper.

Ahava describes an even greater closeness. The
companionship of *ra'ah* is based on acceptance. *Ahava*
goes beyond mere acceptance to commitment. Chandler
illustrates *ahava* like this: It is, he says, when one
partner says, "I don't want to be anywhere else but right
here—right now—with you." But not in the romantic,
watching-the-sun-set-at-the-beach-together sense. No,
ahava is more like when your mate is throwing dishes at
you, and as you dodge them, you're thinking, "I wouldn't
want to be anywhere else but here, dodging the dishes
you're throwing at me. I'm not going anywhere." That's
ahava commitment. When things are terrible, I'm
committed to us. Commitment means being willing to be
unhappy as long as it takes to fix the problem.

It's that kind of *ahava* commitment that, for a
husband and wife, leads to the Hebrew *dod*, the
intermingling of souls. In the context of total acceptance
and commitment, a couple is free to share the deepest and
most vulnerable parts of themselves.

Dod, though closely related to sex, actually means the
soul connection marriage partners are meant to enjoy.
The physical nature of sex is the concrete picture of the

soul connection marriage partners are meant to enjoy. Sex, as God intended it, is the physical expression of *dod*, not just skin-on-skin, but soul-to-soul. *Dod* cements you together.

These different ever-deepening Hebrew words for intimacy show us that God created a progression of deepening closeness. *Ra'ah* leads to *ahava* leads to *dod*. Companionship leads to commitment leads to sex. This is God's process for developing oneness in a couple. Sex is the deepest, most beautiful culmination of intimacy designed to complete God's process, not to begin it.[38]

> **God has a process for developing intimacy—sex is at the END of that process.**

Sex. Technically, sexual intercourse is the insertion of the penis inside the vagina, generally followed by ejaculation. Less technical and more holistically (and better for our purpose), sex is the "physical expression of love and pleasure." It may or may not include intercourse, ejaculation, or orgasm.[39] Sex is God's greatest catalyst for marital oneness. It is the most powerful unifying act there is between a husband & wife.

Sex is Part of "All Things"

The enemy often paints the picture of sex as dirty or wrong. Justin Taylor's argument can retrain our thinking. He points out that sex is a subset of "all things" that God created, so whatever God's Word says about "all things" applies to sex. Consider these truths:

- Sex is created by God. ("By Him *all things* were created," Col. 1:16.)

---

[38] Thanks to Matt Chandler, pastor of The Village Church in Texas, for these definitions. His message series, "Sex," is excellent, available at thevillagechurch.net.
[39] William Cutrer, and Sandra Glahn, *Sexual Intimacy in Marriage* (Grand Rapids, MI: Kregel Publications, 1998), 20.

- Sex continues to exist by the will of Christ. ("In Him *all things* hold together," Col. 1:17.)
- Sex is caused by God. (He "works *all things* together by the counsel of His will," Eph. 1:11.)
- Sex is subject to Christ. ("He put *all things* under His feet," Eph. 1:22.)
- Christ is making sex new. ("Behold, I am making *all things* new," Rev. 21:5.)
- Sex is good. ("*Everything* created by God is good," 1 Tim. 4:4.)
- Sex is lawful in the context of marriage. ("*All things* are lawful," 1 Cor. 10:23.)
- When we have sex, we are to do it for the glory of God. ("*Whatever* you do, do *all* to the glory of God," 1 Cor. 10:31.)
- Sex works together for the good of God's children. ("For those who love God *all things* work together for good, for those who are called according to his purpose," Rom. 8:28.)
- We are to thank God for sex. ("*Nothing* is to be rejected if it is received with thanksgiving," 1 Tim. 4:4.)
- Sex is to be sanctified by the Word of God and prayer. ("*Everything*...is made holy by the Word of God and prayer," 1 Tim. 4:4.)
- We are to be content in sex. ("Having all contentment in *all things* at all times," 2 Cor. 9:8.)
- In this fallen age, sex is both pure and impure. ("To the pure, *all things* are pure, but to the defiled and unbelieving, nothing is pure; but both their minds and their consciences are defiled," Tit. 1:15.)[40]

These verses bring sex out of the gutter and into the light, don't they?

Six Purposes of Sex

God created sex, and it has at least six Heaven-ordained purposes:

---

[40] John Piper and Justin Taylor, ed., *Sex and the Supremacy of Christ* (Wheaton, IL: Crossway Books, 2005), 12-13. Some of Taylor's bullets are left out.

1. Children. God gave Adam and Eve a "Great Commission" before the Fall: "Be fruitful and multiply, fill the earth and subdue it."[41] He wanted to populate the earth with His image bearers. This is a high and holy calling—only rightly fulfilled when there is sex between a husband and wife.

2. Oneness. Sex is intended to make couples one, the core value of marriage.[42] Everything about it is meant to draw one man and one woman into profound closeness. Did you know that humans are the only mammals whose primary sexual position is face-to-face?[43] Even the vulnerability of sex and nakedness are designed to build closeness between committed partners, not to mention the shared pleasure of endorphins that flood lovers' brains.

In fact, the marvelous and complex chemical system behind sex serves to bond a couple together like nothing else in the world. Oxytocin, most well-known as a substance that bonds breastfeeding mothers to their babies, also washes through the brain during sex. It works in both men and women to bond partners together and create feelings of trust. Drs. McIlhaney and Bush say, "the hormonal effect of oxytocin is ideal for marriage."[44]

A great myth is that for a man sex is just about physical pleasure. Not so! Myths and stereotypes are lies from the father of lies meant to divide us. Men need and crave the emotional oneness that comes from sex with their wives, too. If you don't believe me, ask your husband.

3. Knowledge. Nobody knows you like someone you share sex with. It's even reflected in the biblical language:

---

[41] Genesis 1:28.
[42] Genesis 2:24.
[43] Matt Chandler. "Sex." Sermon, The Village Church, Denton, TX, May 15, 2005.
[44] Joe McIlhaney, MD, and Freda McKissic Bush, MD, *Hooked: New Science on How Casual Sex is Affecting Our Children* (Chicago: Northfield Publishing, 2008), 38. We'll consider the chemistry of sex more when we talk about why God reserves it for marriage.

"Adam knew Eve his wife."[45] Sex causes you to be vulnerable and trusting with one other person. God designed sex to be a blessing, allowing you to know your spouse in such an intimate way.

4. *Protection.* 1 Corinthians 7:5 warns, "come together again so that Satan will not tempt you because of your lack of self-control." We'll look at this passage more in depth later, but for now, it is clear that marital sex is a cure for temptation to sin.

5. *Comfort.* When David and Bathsheba's child died as a result of David's sin, he "comforted his wife Bathsheba, and he went to her and lay with her."[46] Sometimes sex offers comfort in a way mere words can't. God designed it for that purpose. Life been tough, lately? Don't neglect the blessing of comfort sex with your mate, and don't withhold that blessing if your partner needs it.

6. *Pleasure.* Last (but not least!), sex is for pleasure! Scientists generally agree that orgasm and the "makes you feel good" nature of sex is not necessary for procreation.[47] Consider some of the intricacies of this marvelous physiological system that works in concert to create the most pleasurable experience known to man.

Chemical messengers are sent to the penis in response to nerve stimulation (or sexual thoughts). These messengers relax smooth muscle in the penis, allowing blood to fill the corpora cavernosa tissue like a balloon. There is connective tissue that keeps blood from flowing out of the penis, giving the penis a significantly higher blood pressure than the rest of a man's body. Then, there's the enzyme in the penis that breaks down the chemical messengers, ensuring that things go back to normal after a short time (end of the erection). A similar blood flow process is going on in the vagina.

---

[45] Genesis 4:1.

[46] 2 Samuel 12:24.

[47] Barry R. Komisaruk, Carlos Beyer-Flores, and Beverly Whipple, *The Science of Orgasm* (Baltimore, MD: Johns Hopkins University Press, 2006), 10.

All the sexual organs are designed with function beyond mere utility. The clitoris' sole purpose is to increase a woman's pleasure during sex. The penis is packed with nerves, all to make sex feel good. But the pleasure of sex is not just in the skin.

Endorphins and other hormones washing the brain during sex make it the highest chemical reward our bodies receive. Some of God's greatest design and engineering have been focused on creating a concert of pleasure. Romantic, intoxicating sex, stress-relief sex, mood-changing sex—God intended it for pleasure.

Sex is a physical, emotional, and spiritual soul connection with the person you care most about in the world. It is a good God who envisioned giving the greatest earthly joy to even the poorest people on earth. Sex is for pleasure—God is good!

Physiology Matters

This is not a book about physiology or technique, but don't underestimate them, either. Though we live in an enlightened, information-rich age, many couples do not understand how their bodies work. Myths abound about how sex is supposed to work.

Contrary to popular belief, most couples do not regularly orgasm simultaneously, and that's okay. If a wife does not experience orgasm regularly, it is worth it to consult your doctor (or at least a good book[48]) and make sure that you understand the basic mechanics.

It is not uncommon for couples to have been so shy with each other that they are missing what sex is designed to be. What a tragedy to be one discovery away

---

[48] There are several good books mentioned in the resources, but *Sexual Intimacy in Marriage* (written by an M.D.) is particularly good regarding misunderstood mechanics.

from exponentially greater joy. You have to learn what works for each of you. You need to communicate through this process. If talking about sex has been hard for you, you've come to the right place! Keep reading.

Finally, don't neglect good health, either. Exercise and vitamins can make a tremendous difference for the better if you're not feeling good about sex emotionally or physically. Depression can decrease sex drive dramatically. Seek the aid of a physician or psychiatrist if libido is affected beyond a few weeks.

Walk Through the Bible

God has not been silent about what He intended for sex. Scripture outlines a complete theology of intimacy. Examining foundational passages on marriage (e.g., Ephesians 5:25-35 and 1 Corinthians 13) or a complete study of the Song of Solomon, while eminently fruitful for any couple, would broaden our subject too much to keep us focused on how to lead to the bedroom.

To stay on track, we're going to delve into seven foundational passages specifically about God's design for sexual intimacy. Looking at these passages in Bible order presents them roughly in order of the progress of revelation. Perhaps we should call this section *Everything you ever wanted to know about sex, but didn't think you'd read in the Bible.*

Genesis 2-3: God's Original Design

Since we've already examined extensively (in the last chapter) God's original intent when he created Adam and Eve, let's just briefly review principles from Genesis 2:

- *Marriage is meant to be a helping relationship.*[49]

---
[49] Genesis 2:18.

- *Oneness is the core value of marriage.* That's what God designed it for: "Two shall become one flesh."[50]

- *Openness and complete vulnerability is God's intent.* The first couple were "naked and not ashamed."[51]

- *The wife is the husband's standard of beauty (and vice versa).* Making the first couple as a pair with no odd man (or woman) out indicates that God never intended a beauty contest where a man compares the beauty of his partner with others.[52] Scripture affirms this in one of the qualifications of an elder: he is to be a "one-woman man."[53]

- *Satan wants to destroy the oneness God gave.*[54] Therefore, we need to be careful to avoid his lies.

Proverbs 5: Under the Influence

Solomon, the wisest man who ever lived, gives us his first counsel regarding sexual intimacy in Proverbs 5:15-20:

*15 Drink water from **your own** cistern,*
*running water from **your own** well.*

God gave you your own wife to satisfy your sexual thirst. She is yours; when you are thirsty, have a drink.

16 Should your springs overflow in the streets,

---

[50] Genesis 2:24.
[51] Genesis 2:25.
[52] Driscoll. "The Peasant Princess." Sermon series, Mars Hill Church, Seattle, WA, September-October, 2008.
[53] 1 Timothy 3:2.
[54] Genesis 3:7 and John 10:10.

your streams of water in the public squares?
17 Let them be yours alone,
never to be shared with strangers.
18 May your fountain be blessed,
and may you rejoice in the wife of your youth.

Solomon compares a wife's sexuality to a private spring meant only for one man. She is not to be shared with strangers, but is always to be a delight to her husband alone. Husband, he says, rejoice that you've got the blessing of a wife who can satisfy you sexually.

19 A loving doe, a graceful deer—
may her breasts satisfy you always, may you ever
*be **captivated** by her **love**.*

Deer are gentle and beautiful animals—and easily frightened. Solomon is saying a man is to approach his wife gently.[55] He shifts from metaphor to actual: "Let her breasts satisfy you always."

The Bible is clear that Christians should never be drunk, but under the control of the Holy Spirit.[56] However, there is one more thing we are strongly encouraged to be "under the influence" of—our sexual relationship with our spouse. Proverbs 5:19b says, "May you ever be captivated by her love."

"Captivated" means "exhilarated" or "intoxicated." In context, "her love" is the sexual relationship. Solomon compares kissing and sex to wine at least twice in the Song of Solomon (see Song 4:10 and 7:9). Too much wine makes you do strange things—and want it more. Solomon says sex with your one and only wife has a similar effect, and it's a wise thing for you to be under its influence.

---

[55] Tommy Nelson, *The Song of Solomon: A Study of Love, Sex, Marriage and Romance*, VHS (Dallas, TX: Hudson Productions, 1995).
[56] Ephesians 5:18.

20 Why be captivated, my son, by an adulteress?
Why embrace the bosom of another man's wife?

The word "adulteress" is literally a "foreigner"—one you don't know. Solomon says, "You've got everything you need!" It would be foolish to go after another man's wife. Anyone who commits adultery ultimately comes to the same conclusion. Too bad Solomon's own heart did not heed his wise counsel.

Song of Solomon: The Greatest Song

Do you like chick flicks? I mean, a really great love story. Most films these days have a romantic, passionate sex scene where the young lovers are enraptured with each other and lose themselves in the passion and pleasure of enjoying each other. Even while we're trying not to watch, we often look at our own marriages and sigh that the movie's portrayal of love is unrealistic.

However, the Song of Solomon, the crown jewel of God's Word on sexual intimacy, paints a passionate and erotic picture beyond what any film could ever capture. This three-thousand-year-old love story has never been more relevant than today.

God didn't reveal all of His truth in propositions, commands, and prohibitions. Most of the Bible, in fact, is narrative (story). God has given us some direct instructions about sex, this great catalyst for oneness He created. But when He wanted to illustrate what it is meant to look like, He didn't use dogma or commands—He gave us a story.

Solomon, the wisest man who ever lived, who had all the money, power, and fame life could offer, was led by God to write his greatest poem about...wait for it—loving one woman with all his heart and her loving him and them giving themselves to each other completely.

His "greatest song"[57] is a love "song" (series of poems) which tells the story of the courtship, wedding, honeymoon, and deepening marriage (including a fight and resolution) of King Solomon and his bride. A complete study would fill a book in itself, so here I'll just outline three broad principles.[58] Find an overview of the book in Figure 4.

Figure 4.
Outline of the Song of Solomon

Section	Phase	Description
1:1-3:5	Attraction & Courtship	Includes the excitement, passion, pursuit, insecurities, fears, reassurance, and restraint of a relationship before marriage
3:6 – 4:1	Wedding Ceremony	Includes the pomp and celebration of the big day, highlighting the beauty and value of the bride and celebrating that the wait is over
4:1-5:1	Honeymoon	Most erotic passage in the Scriptures; God gives His stamp of approval on passionate sex in marriage
5:2 – 8:14	Maturing Marriage	Includes conflict, resolution (even closer than before), keeping romance and passion alive, and gratefulness to God for a loving relationship

The first truth illustrated in the Song to emphasize for our theology of intimacy is that *the husband is to lead his wife into intimacy.* Solomon says to his bride,

Arise, my darling, my beautiful one, and come with me. See! The winter is past; the rains are over

---

[57] Song 1:1; The "Song of Songs" means the song that stands out above all other songs...the greatest song.
[58] Understanding the entire *Song* is a very profitable study for your marriage. For help interpreting it, see several resources listed in the back of the book and at leadingtothebedroom.com.

*and gone. Flowers appear on the earth; the season
of singing has come, the cooing of doves is heard in
our land.*[59]

God created marriage (all human spheres, actually:
church, government, labor, family) with a leader. If the
husband doesn't lead, then other forces in your life will.
The busyness of life will consume you, and you will miss
out on a passionate love life. This effective enemy tactic
by the thief counts on the husband not leading.
Remember what happened in Genesis 3 when Adam
remained silent? Don't fall prey to his scheme. Solomon
led his bride to greater intimacy in their relationship. The
rest of this book is about how to do that.

Here's the second principle: *Tenderness +
Responsiveness = Satisfaction.* Solomon teaches us that
God's design for marital love is intended to be
uninhibited, mutually pleasing, and erotic. In the book,
the couple isn't perfect, but they are completely
committed to each other and to nurturing their
relationship. Sex plays a huge role in their relationship. A
recurring pattern is that the husband's tenderness
coupled with his wife's responsiveness yields satisfaction
and joy in their relationship.

Solomon's third truth for our theology of intimacy is
that *God has stamped His seal of approval on passionate,
erotic sex in marriage.* The honeymoon, Solomon and his
bride's first sexual encounter described in Song 4:1-5:1, is
filled with tender and erotic words. The bride invites her
husband into "his" garden to taste choice fruit. Solomon
does so, and then with a satiated sigh announces,

*I have come into my garden, my sister, my bride; I
have gathered my myrrh with my spice. I have*

---

[59] Song of Solomon 2:10-12.

eaten my honeycomb and my honey; I have drunk my wine and my milk.[60]

Solomon uses several images to describe intimacy with his bride. She is a garden (a refreshing oasis), myrrh with spice (a sweet-smelling luxury), and honey, wine, and milk (sweet and nourishing food and drink). Also, don't miss how many times he refers to her as "mine." Sex is meant to bond spouses together like that.

But it's what happens next that is utterly remarkable! Another voice speaks up in the honeymoon bedroom.

"Eat, O friends, and drink; drink your fill, O lovers."[61]

God Himself says eat up and drink up.[62] Enjoy each other fully. The refrain of the book up until this point, "Do not arouse or awaken love until it is time,"[63] was for before marriage. I love it that our God is for passionate, ear-ringing marital sex! "Enjoy each other with My blessing, God says. "That's what I made it for! Go for it!" Wow! This has got to be one of my favorite verses in God's Word.

---

[60] Song of Solomon 5:1a.

[61] Song of Solomon 5:1b.

[62] Some attribute these words to the daughters of Jerusalem (the bride's friends). However, practically, they wouldn't be in the honeymoon chamber. But more important, theologically, God saying "eat and drink" perfectly fits the message of the book. In Chapter 8, we find out it is God who has been guiding them before they knew each other and brought them together. He would be the one in the honeymoon suite saying, "This is good and right. Enjoy each other to the fullest."

[63] Song 2:7 and 3:5. The exhortation is repeated in 8:4 (after the wedding), but then it is said to the daughters of Jerusalem to encourage them to save sex until marriage because it was worth the wait.

A Wife's Take

For a girl who grew up with a heart for God and a great background of godly encouragement to wait until marriage, it was hard to turn 22 years of teaching that (premarital) sex is wrong into "go for it." In the Song of Solomon, God gives us a picture of it. The refrain, "Do not arouse or awaken love until it pleases" is repeated until the honeymoon. Then, the restraint is cast off, and God says to enjoy each other fully. Sex was not wrong before, it was just "not now."

John 2: Shame Turned to Joy

In my Christian circles growing up, Jesus turning water into wine in John 2 was taught as demonstrating the miraculous power of Jesus, proving His divinity at the very outset of His ministry. On a less glorious note, the passage also figured prominently in the debate over whether consuming alcohol was a sin.

While the first is certainly true, and the latter is not my subject, both miss the real point Jesus was making about why He came. John 2:11 calls this event "the first of Jesus' miraculous *signs*." A sign always points to a deeper truth beyond itself.

His first miracle, transforming water into wine, was His statement to the world, a sign, that He was coming to transform our relationship with God. He chose water, which is mundane and tasteless, to represent the law, which by itself is not a joyful way to relate to God. And He replaced it with wine, a symbol of joy and abundance. Through His first miracle, Jesus showed that His purpose was to bring us a great, joyful life with God. The details of the story give us more insight into His mission.

The host was responsible to provide guests with wine for seven days, the duration of the wedding celebration. To fail on this account would be shameful. Jesus' intervention at just the right time removed the shame that was certain to befall the groom. It's a beautiful picture of the gospel. Jesus wasn't responsible for the groom's shame, but He took it upon Himself to remove it. The grace Jesus showed was a glimpse of His entire mission to take away humanity's shame.

Jesus didn't make just enough wine, He made an abundance—six stone water pots holding about thirty gallons each! He was showing us that His grace is plentiful—almost absurdly so. And don't miss the master of ceremonies' comment: "You have saved the best wine until now."[64] What Jesus has to bring us is the best!

What Jesus has to bring us is the best!

Now think about the context. Jesus performed His first miracle—at a wedding! The good news of Christ permeates every area of our lives. In the beginning, God instituted marriage as soon as He created man. Marriage was God's first and greatest blessing for His new creation. Later, when Jesus came to set everything right that the enemy destroyed, He, too, began with a statement—a sign—about marriage: I've come to restore it (along with everything else) to its original state of unashamed joy and abundance. That's good news!

In John 2, Jesus is sending couples a message. I've come to bring life and joy and to set right all that has gone wrong in marriage since the Fall. Whatever the state of your marriage, don't give up. You can experience the gospel in your marriage.

---

[64] John 2:10.

1 Corinthians 7: Stop Robbing Each Other

A longitudinal secular study concluded that 15% of Americans are having 50% of the sex.[65] Forget the veracity of the study (or how they gathered their data), but think about this question: does more sex translate into a better marriage?

Before we devolve into a *men say yes/women say no* division, let's consider 1 Corinthians 7:1-9:

> *1 Now for the matters you wrote about: It is good for a man not to marry.*

Whoa, whoa, whoa, hold up—Paul, the man who penned Ephesians 5:22-32, says marriage is bad?! God Himself said, "It is not good for the man to be alone."

Context and careful interpretation are needed. "To marry" carries the translation too far. Literally, Paul's statement in the Greek is, "It is good for a man not to *touch a woman.*" This was a euphemism for intercourse, and according to all the teaching of the Bible, would imply marriage. Put simply, Paul is saying celibacy (for a single) is a good thing. He goes on to imply in verse 26 and verse 29 that his advice on celibacy (it it good not to take a wife) is specifically because of "this present distress." This was probably persecution against the church that could make it difficult to keep the faith if you had a wife and kids because you might be forced to choose between their safety and living for the gospel.

Verse one was also perhaps the Corinthians' question to him, something along the lines of "Are you saying a man should never be with a woman sexually?" Paul's answer: "Celibacy (and not taking a wife) is a good thing, especially during this present distress, but..." (Continue to verse two.)

---

[65] John Student, "No Sex, Please...We're College Graduates," *American Demographics*, February 1998, 31.

2 But since there is so much immorality, each man should have his own wife, and each woman her own husband.

The implication here is that marital sex is a tool of God to prevent sin.

3 The husband should fulfill his marital duty to his wife, and likewise the wife to her husband.
4 The wife's body does not belong to her alone but also to her husband. In the same way, the husband's body does not belong to him alone but also to his wife.

Your body now has mutual ownership. It no longer belongs to you alone but also to your spouse. You have a duty to be intimate with your spouse when he or she needs it. That is God's intent with your sexuality and partnership.

5 Do not <u>deprive</u> each other...

The Greek verb *apostereo* means "to cause another to suffer loss by taking something away through illicit means." Its synonyms are rob, steal, and defraud. In its present active imperative form, literally, Paul is saying, "Stop robbing each other!"

...except by <u>mutual</u> consent and for a <u>time</u>, so <u>that you may devote yourselves to prayer</u>.

Then, Paul lays out what I believe are the normal spiritual conditions under which a couple would be right to abstain. This means that the default position in marriage is that both partners are there for each other. Here are the conditions for abstinence:

1) "mutual consent"—you've <u>both</u> decided to abstain for a specific reason

2) "for a time"—this means a short, defined time period—not long or open-ended.

3) "so that you may devote yourselves to prayer"— sometimes there will be something so big that you need to pray about that you as a couple decide "we need to hear from God so badly on this that we are going to abstain so that we can fully seek His direction."[66]

Biblically speaking, you should not deprive each other unless you have both decided to fast from sex (for a short time) in order to seek God.

> *Then come together again so that Satan will not tempt you because of your lack of self-control.*

Notice that Paul adds a warning about abstaining: come together again so Satan will not tempt you. Abstaining from sex when you are married is a dangerous place to be. The enemy will try to tempt you. The cure to sexual temptation is to have sex often with your spouse.

The cure to sexual temptation is to have sex often with your spouse.

> *6 I say this as a concession, not as a command. 7 I wish that all men were as I am. But each man has his own gift from God; one has this gift, another has that. 8 Now to the unmarried and the widows I say: It is good for them to stay unmarried, as I am.*

Implication: Some men (or women) need sex more than others. One person has the gift of celibacy; another has a different gift. Again, verse 8 reflects Paul's view of

---

[66] The purpose of fasting is to get rid of all distractions and to put seeking Him first before our own comfort.

the world in Corinth. Because of persecution, it's better to stay single if you are not married right now.[67]

9 But if they cannot control themselves, they should marry, for it is better to marry than to burn with passion.

Implication: The marriage relationship is God's answer for a high sex drive. Again, Paul makes it clear that if you are married, you should be able to be satisfied sexually—that's God's design.

The frequency of sex among many couples today is dangerously low. Paul says if you have a spouse, that should not be the case. Husbands and wives need to recognize that the only way each partner can legitimately meet his or her needs for sexual release is through relationship with one's spouse.

Don't give the enemy a foothold by withholding the one thing that can keep your spouse from being tempted sexually. Scripture says the cure to temptation is to have sex with your spouse often.[68]

This begs important questions: Does this mean you can never say no? Does this give a husband or wife the right to be selfish or demanding? We will consider frequency and ways to meet both partners' needs in depth later in the book,[69] but for now let me just encourage husband and wife that 1 Corinthians 7:1-9 should be lived out by each partner in the spirit of *agape* love (1 Cor. 13) and 1 Peter 3:7:

7 Husbands, in the same way be considerate as you live with your wives, and treat them with

---

[67] Singleness is a gift from God that allows you to do many things for the sake of the gospel that married people can't. If you have that gift from God, leverage it for the Kingdom.

[68] 1 Corinthians 7:5.

[69] See Chapter Seven if you can't wait for the answer.

respect as the weaker partner and as heirs with you of the gracious gift of life, so that nothing will hinder your prayers.

Husband, never forget that your wife is the daughter of the King. Do not mistreat her.

Hebrews 13:4: The Marriage Bed is Pure

Scripture's rundown of Christian behavior in Hebrews 13 highlights the value God places on the exclusivity on the marriage relationship. Here's verse four:

Marriage should be honored by all, and the marriage bed kept pure, for God will judge the adulterer and all the sexually immoral.

The marriage bed (symbolic for the sexual relationship in marriage) is pure. It should not be defiled by sharing that gift outside of marriage, for God will judge those who use this pure gift for marriage outside of that relationship.

It is significant that God tells us sex in marriage is pure. Genesis 2 showed us that marriage by God's design was without shame, the Song of Solomon illustrated the freedom and passion possible (and encouraged) for sex in marriage, and Hebrews 13:4 adds that this is pure in God's sight. That means this gift for oneness is NOT defiling or unclean or unacceptable to God, as long as it is in marriage for the purpose of oneness. Want to try different positions, locations, or ways of pleasuring your spouse? Go ahead, experiment! The marriage bed is pure.

What is Forbidden—and Why

As a co-op (work/study) student at Georgia Tech, I moved in and out of the dorm every other quarter. Over five years, I had more than fifteen college roommates (that will give you good preparation for cooperation in marriage). On one occasion, my roommate had a male and a female friend who hung out frequently in our dorm room. These friends of his began dating, became sexually active, and then she broke up with him all within the course of a school quarter.

The crushed guy crashed in our dorm (lucky us!) as he agonized the night away with primal screams of pain I have never forgotten. I've often wished I could play his screams for our church as a warning. He had connected his soul to a woman without the security of commitment. God never intended such pain for His creation.

Within marriage, God leaves the door wide open for sex. Outside of marriage, He closes it tight, and by doing so, He protects us from such pain. Paul forbids sexual activity outside God's intended plan in 1 Corinthians 6:18a:

Flee immorality.

God's people aren't usually told to run from things in the Bible. Giants? Face them with faith. Meat offered to idols? Eat it with a clear conscience. Strongholds? Tear them down with God's power. But *porneia* (sexual immorality)—run away from it!

Porneia (the Greek word translated "immorality" in this verse) is a catch-all term. It means anything that is sinful in the sexual arena. Here's a list of things prohibited sexually in the Scriptures:

Sexual Immorality God Prohibits

Adultery – voluntary sex between a married person and someone other than his or her spouse (Ex. 20:14)
Bestiality – sex with animals (Lev. 18:23)

Bisexuality – sex with both man and woman (Lev. 18:22; Rom. 1:26-27)

Fornication – sexual acts outside marriage, including masturbation used as a tool for lust (Eph. 5:3; 1 Thess. 4:1-8)

Homosexuality – sex with someone of the same sex (Lev. 18:22; Rom. 1:26-27)

Incest – sex with a close relative (Lev. 18:6-18)

Lust –misdirected desire for sexual stimulation; to want what God has not given you (Ex. 20:17; Eph. 5:3-5)

Pedophilia – sexual perversion in which children are the preferred object (Gen. 2:21-25; Matt. 7:12)

Polygamy – marriage in which a spouse may have more than one mate at the same time (Gen. 2:21-25)

Pornography – viewing materials that depict erotic images or behavior to cause immoral sexual excitement (Job 31:1) *This would include sexual chatting with someone other than your spouse.*

Prostitution – engaging in sex for money or false worship (Deut. 23:17-18; 1 Cor. 6:18-20)

Rape – sex carried out forcefully against one's will (Gen. 2:21-25; Matt. 7:12)

Paul provides an intriguing explanation for why God says to run from these things. It's in the second half of 1 Corinthians 6:18:

Every other sin that a man commits is outside the body, but the immoral man [one committing sexual immorality][70] *sins against his own body.*

Porneia, Paul says, is a sin against one's own body compared to every other sin. Not trusting God with your

---

[70] The Greek participle here is from the verb *porneuo* (same root as *porneia*) and means "one who commits sexual immorality." It, too, is a catch-all term designating any type of sexual sin.

life, sinful money management, gluttony, drug abuse, even suicide—all have effects on the human body, but Paul says *porneia* is in a category all by itself. With sexual sin, there is a qualitative difference in terms of the destructiveness of its effects on your self. What is that difference?

Once I heard a minister describe marital oneness in a wedding sermon as similar to the bonding that happens when a tongue is stuck to a frozen flagpole. The two become one, and to separate them is the worst kind of pain. It's not the most romantic image, but it illustrates Paul's point. When you bond sexually with someone or something outside of God's plan, you're hurting yourself in the worst kind of way. Our bodies were designed for oneness with one other human being in marriage. Everything God forbids in the catch-all *porneia* are things that lead away from this oneness between a married husband and wife that God intended.

Science Confirms It

The more we learn, the more medical science confirms what Paul said two thousand years ago. During sex, the brain is washed with hormones. Three of them in particular were designed by God specifically to make sex a bonding experience between a married man and woman. The work of these chemicals confirm that God has designed sex as the greatest catalyst for oneness between two people committed in marriage.

Oxytocin. We've already mentioned oxytocin, most well-known as a substance that bonds breastfeeding mothers to their babies. It's released during breastfeeding and it has the effect of bonding a woman with someone she touches. This is a beautiful and needed system, considering that seven-pound newborn just caused the mother the worst physical pain she's ever had. But as oxytocin is released, all pain is forgotten, and the love between mother and child is cemented.

Oxytocin is also released when a woman is touched in a loving way, and even more during intercourse. It has a similar bonding effect toward a man when released during intimacy. Consider Drs. McIlhaney and Bush's sobering words:

> [The chemical reaction of bonding from oxytocin] is an involuntary process that cannot distinguish between a one-night stand and a lifelong soul mate. Oxytocin can cause a woman to bond to a man even during what was expected to be a short-term sexual relationship. So when that short-term relationship ends, the emotional fallout can be devastating, thanks to oxytocin.[71]

This sheds a whole new light on "the one committing sexual immorality sins against his own body," doesn't it?

Dopamine. Thank God for dopamine! This neurotransmitter makes you feel exhilarated when it is pumped through your brain. It works as a reward signal—you feel a rush when it's flowing. When you take a risk, it flows to reward you for taking that risk. The kicker is that dopamine is values-neutral—you can feel that rush whether you witness for Christ or you steal a car.

Dopamine floods your brain during sex. No matter how bad things seem, you can have sex with your spouse and all is right with the world again. Comfort sex has a chemical basis—God made it that way to bless us.

But since it's values-neutral, you feel that same rush if you have sex without the security of commitment. That's a very dangerous place to be. Unfortunately, teens who experience premarital sex find that dopamine rush from sex an almost irresistible urge. *The immoral man sins against his own body.*

---

[71] McIlhaney and Bush, *Hooked*, 45.

Vasopressin. This male hormone washes the male brain during intercourse. It causes him to feel bonded to a woman he is intimate with. God's design is that the first act of sex on the wedding night bonds the groom to his bride in a way he's never been bonded with another woman ("the two shall become one flesh") and every encounter after that "till death do us part" serves to deepen that bond.

Multiple partners, and even attaching to pornography via masturbation, can weaken the ability of a man to emotionally bond with one person. McIlhaney and Bush compare it to tape that loses its stickiness when it is continually applied and removed. Vasopressin was doing its job in my college roommate's friend. He bonded to a woman without the security of commitment.

Sexual intimacy outside God's plan foils the marvelous chemical system God designed to bond us and bless us. With these powerful sexual hormones hard at work during each sexual encounter to bond you to your marriage partner, it's no wonder Paul said, "let there not be even a hint of sexual immorality among you."[72] He didn't know the neurochemistry behind 1 Corinthians 6:18—but God did, and He led Paul to warn us:

> *Flee immorality. Every other sin that a man commits is outside the body, but the immoral man sins against his own body.*

Protection and Provision

Every command God gives is to protect and provide for you. He wants to make sex in marriage the best it can be to bless you and to protect you. It was designed to deepen that relationship and that relationship alone.

---

[72] Ephesians 5:3.

All the things that God has forbidden sexually are things that do not promote oneness between a married couple. This is what God designed sex for. For example, God commands us not to lust. Looking at pornography is a form of lusting. Viewing pornography is NOT helpful to your marriage. It violates your wife being your standard of beauty.[73] It puts you in danger of bonding sexually with images other than your wife.[74] This defeats God's purpose of oneness for you and your spouse (or future spouse if you're single). Therefore, God prohibits it to protect you. If you take the fire out of the fireplace, it's dangerous, and you can get hurt—in fact, you can burn the whole house down.

Conversely—and this is great news!—anything that promotes marital oneness is allowed. One problem many couples have after marriage (those who waited as well as those who were promiscuous before marriage) is this: *after* you're married, it's hard to flip that switch that kept you pure (or convicted you of promiscuity[75]) before the wedding. So, what does healthy married sex look like, or put another way, what is okay in bed? Anything that brings about oneness in your marriage.

The guidelines of Christian *Real Sex* columnists Melissa and Louis McBurney[76] are illuminating. They advocate that married sex should be:

Exclusive – It is only for husband and wife (no others involved).

---

[73] Genesis 2:22-25, Song of Solomon 1.

[74] Douglas Weiss, *Sex, Men, & God: A Godly Man's Roadmap to Sexual Success* (Lake Mary, FL: Siloam, 2002), 18.

[75] Feeling guilty for past sexual sin? God is a God who forgives and casts our sin into the "depths of the sea" (Micah 7:19). Isn't that a beautiful way of saying He doesn't hold our sin against us? Ask God and your mate for forgiveness, and walk in freedom from the past.

[76] Unfortunately, *Marriage Partnership* magazine (where their column appeared) is out of print. But many of its articles and the *Real Sex* column live on at ChristianityToday.com. Read the full article, *Christian Sex Rules*, at www.christianitytoday.com/mp/2001/spring/4.34.html?start=1.

Mutual – Both partners sacrifice their own needs for what they can agree on to mutually benefit the other. Frequency, romance, and experimentation are all on the table to promote the greatest oneness. Anything that hurts, demeans, or makes either partner feel hurt or demeaned should be avoided.

Pleasurable – Anything that causes harm or pain goes against the oneness God intended.

Relational – Sex is meant to be soul-on-soul, not just skin-on-skin. All your sexual activity should be increasing your relational intimacy.

Perpetuating Genital Union – Obviously, God's primary sexual position design is face-to-face, penis-in-vagina. All the parts just fit. This guideline simply means don't neglect this primary position for long. It is the epitome of exclusive, mutual, pleasurable, and relational.

Other than avoiding what is forbidden and valuing these broad principles of oneness, husband and wife are completely free to enjoy the adventure, passion, discovery, eroticism, ecstasy, and beauty of sex. God says,

"Eat, O friends, and drink; drink your fill, O lovers."[77]

Welcome to Soul Sex

In short, God intended frequent, playful, erotic, and sensual sex to be a tool to build marital oneness. God created us for soul sex—a three-dimensional spiritual, emotional, and physical connection meant to bond us together so much that we will be faithful and bless each other for a lifetime. This chemical/physical/soul activity strengthens our marriage bond through hard seasons of life and brings a climax of joy to the best of days. It gives expression to inexpressible love throughout marriage.

---

[77] Song of Solomon 5:1b.

Men were created to be pursuers, leaders, wife-desirers. That's why we brim with testosterone. Women were created to be responders, eager and willing to engage their loving husbands, showing them respect (his greatest need) and care by giving themselves fully and frequently to their husbands.

Soul sex with his wife makes a husband feel powerful and virile. A wife feels beautiful and treasured when she connects at a soul level with her husband. The beauty of God's design is stunning—a robust system that meets needs and blesses both partners.

And God meant it to be breath-taking and soul-stirring. Why is exciting, frequent sex more soul stirring that "regular" sex? Men are wired for adventure. God made them that way.[78] Variety, passion, erotic experiments, and adventure reach deeply into a man's heart. Who doesn't want to experience *everything* their marriage has to offer?

Conclusion

Of all the gifts you received at your wedding, one was greater than the rest...the gift that keeps on giving! God Himself gives every married couple, from the wealthiest to the poorest, the lifetime gift of sexual intimacy.

This gift is the grand dessert, a reward for the hard work of cultivating a great marriage day after day.

This gift is a firestarter. It is the greatest catalyst for oneness God has made. Like a fire in your fireplace at home, intimacy can make your marriage warm (and hot, something God created you to desire). But also like that fire, it *must* stay in its proper context, or it can destroy

---

[78] *Wild at Heart* by John Eldredge does a fabulous job of capturing key elements of God's design for men. Eldredge says we were created to live an adventure, fight a battle, and rescue a beauty. Add "for the glory of God" to his tasks, and you've got a great definition of "image bearer."

everything. This gift is one of God's greatest tools to grow you closer together over a lifetime. God intended frequent, playful, erotic, and sensual sex to be a catalyst for married oneness.

It's an incredible gift. Those who value it find it to produce a lifetime of protection, provision, and blessing.

But, there is still the problem identified in Chapter One. The thief came to steal, kill, and destroy the gift God gave. Satan lies, distracts, and shames couples out of the blessing of sexual intimacy, doing everything He can to keep them out of the bedroom.

Because of Satan's deception, Christian wives often inadvertently push their husbands away. As a result of his schemes, Christian husbands often fail to lead to the bedroom (perhaps even thinking they are doing the loving thing). If you are not experiencing soul sex, God's design for His great wedding gift to you, the enemy has succeeded in stealing this precious gift from you.

How does your sex life compare to our theology (God's perspective) of intimacy? Have you lost the passion for sex? Does your spouse secretly wish for more soul connection, either in romance and courting (most often left wanting by the wife), or frequent and erotic sex (most often craved by the husband)? Has the enemy stolen oneness from you? Has he hidden the greatest wedding gift God gave you, the greatest catalyst to increasing oneness that God made for you and your spouse?

Perhaps you're only one degree off course. Things aren't as good as they could be. One degree off course over time will get you totally lost from God's great design for your marriage.

Soul sex is a sexual relationship between husband and wife that stirs your souls and deepens your oneness. Are you fully experiencing it? Or has the enemy stolen it from you?

Christian husbands must take the initiative to lead their wives to the bedroom (and blessing):

by courting

by opening communication

by leading to soul intimacy.

And ladies, you've got to follow and respond to your husband's leadership. You don't want to forfeit the greatest wedding present God has given you. Turn the page to learn how to LEAD to the bedroom.

A Wife's Take

As Dave began to lead us intentionally into deeper intimacy in our marriage, I have to tell you, I've been led way out of my comfort zone. When David began to share what was really in his mind about where he wanted to go in our sex life, I was uncomfortable, even a little fearful at first.

But as I listened to this godly man that God put in my life, who loves me so like Christ loves the church, I also heard from God. What Dave was saying <u>was</u> how it was meant to be.

As we've prayed and persisted, it's become obvious that soul sex is a God thing. I needed to be out of my comfort zone for the sake of our oneness.

Ladies, if your husband takes an active role to lead you toward God's design for intimacy with you, don't shut him down. You'll be glad you didn't!

Chapter Three
From Passive to Passionate
The LEAD Process

Arise, my darling, my beautiful one, and come with me. See! The winter is past; the rains are over and gone.
— The Greatest Song 2:10

The definition of insanity is doing the same thing over and over again and expecting a different result.
— Author Unknown

A Husband's Prayer
Heavenly Father,

I thought I was acting in love by being sensitive to my wife's wishes, but I now realize the MORE loving thing to do is to lead and motivate us into what You created for us to enjoy. I am charged to head our household—to be the leader, to move us toward following Christ.

I take responsibility for us in finances, in parenting, in decisions—in life. I've always felt at peace in that role; You gave it to me, You help me by your wisdom, and You gave me a bride who submits to me as I submit to You.

But somehow, in the role of leading in intimacy, I've really made her take the lead: in frequency, in freedom, in passion. Lord, help me to tenderly, but deliberately, lead us to the next step of sexual intimacy in our marriage.

The Dream

In our heart of hearts, whether man or woman, we all want the deep intimacy, passion, and unselfish love described in Chapter Two. However, because the enemy has been so successful at stealing soul sex, the incredible gift God bestowed on the marriage relationship, most couples are not experiencing the depth and richness of intimacy He intended.

In marriages all over Christendom, wives desperately long for more tenderness, patience, romance, courtship, care, and dad time with the kids. In short, women want their husbands to belong to them more fully. That's every wife's dream. And that's what God intended when He entrusted His daughter to a man.

At the same time, so many Christian husbands all over the world crave more frequent, more fun, more passionate, more soul-stirring sex—in short, they want their wives to belong fully to them.

If you doubt these inner thoughts of your partner, ask your spouse right now if what I've said is true of him or her...I dare you.

One husband put into words for all married men how passionate and free sex increases his feelings of oneness with his wife:

> [Trying this new position] is soul-stirring, it's not my favorite position, because it lacks the face-to-face union we love and need. Why then does it touch my soul at such a deep level?
>
> I think it has an intimacy of its own because of what it represents to me: first, my wife submitted her body, mind, and soul to something she believed I'd like; that's extremely intimate.
>
> Second, it is a new experience; it's something we've never tried; it's fresh; it's another technique in our repertoire to touch each other's souls. It makes a statement of love and selflessness that she is willing to meet my needs.

Finding this [position] together is certainly part of our incredible adventure together for me, and sharing this adventure with her makes me feel close to her like nothing else in the world.

God created the man with more testosterone and a higher sex drive, with a very real felt need for uninhibited, adventurous soul sex with his wife. This is a need for intimacy with his wife—to enjoy her in every way possible.

Ladies, let me tell you what your husband may not have been able to say to you in a long time. Men think about sex with their wives all the time. (I've heard every 17 seconds!) Your husband thinks about sex with you when he wakes up, when you wake up, when he's in the shower, when you're in the shower, when he sees you naked for a moment changing clothes, when he sees you in your bra and panties, when you're putting on your makeup, when you look so pretty dressed for the day, when you smile at him, when you parent, when you give each other a peck on the cheek, when you fix him something to eat for breakfast—and that's all before 7:15 in the morning.[79]

Not only does he think about sex with you all the time, wife, but he desires to have YOU (his own wife, not anyone else) in uninhibited, playful, wild, erotic, romantic, breath-taking, sexy, intimate, experimental, new, exciting, risky (in location), unique, fun, flirtatious, titillating, and sensual ways...not occasionally, but *very* frequently. That kind of freedom is every man's dream. And that's what God intended when He "brought her to the man."[80] Sex is God's greatest catalyst for married oneness.

---

[79] Later, we'll discuss that some men, like women, can have their sexual desires and passions blocked by a variety of saboteurs, but, in general, husbands see the world through sex-colored glasses.
[80] Genesis 2:22.

The Reality

And yet wives often think they are not attractive, wanted, or appreciated. And it's no secret that sex as it's often done in marriage can be a dividing, rather than a uniting, force. How does this happen?

...and yet wives often think they are not attractive, wanted, or appreciated.

Here's the problem. Men don't know how to lead in the sexual arena, wives don't know how to follow, and none of us realize how high the stakes are.

The Soul Sex Pyramid

You see, true soul sex is made up of layers of increasing intimacy. They go from foundational (the bedrock of what makes a Christian marriage) to "icing on the cake"—the soul-stirring and love-giving parts unique to each couple that make sex an indescribable blessing to your relationship.

Typically, the soul sex pyramid looks something like Figure 5. First, for a couple to experience soul sex, the intimacy God intended, there must be *agape* commitment, a selfless loving pledge of faithfulness to each other that provides a secure foundation for vulnerable sexuality to build on.

Then, there's frequency. When one partner asks for sex and is rejected often, he (or she) becomes less likely to ask. Can you see how the enemy steals occasions for oneness when the uncertain, "awkward ask" is in play on a regular basis? (We'll talk more about this later.)

This dynamic makes sex scarce and makes it very difficult to get to more passionate and free stages of expressing intimacy. Only after you solve the issue of low frequency can you move into the higher levels of fun, freedom, and passion, which are all part of the lifelong wedding gift of soul sex God intended in marriage.

Soul sex is everything you read in our theology of intimacy in Chapter Two. (Remember how much Solomon and his bride enjoyed each other?) Perhaps, you may think, some of the higher levels are *merely* icing on the cake—not really necessary for a great marriage. Don't make the mistake of discounting your spouse's needs as less important than your own.[81] This goes for husbands and wives and for areas outside of sex.

Besides, who doesn't want the icing on the cake? Unlike sugary dessert, there's nothing detrimental about indulging in sex. In fact, it's good for you **Who doesn't want the icing on the cake?** emotionally, physically, and maritally. I don't know about you, but I don't want the thief stealing *anything* God gave us in marriage.

Figure 5.
The Soul Sex Pyramid

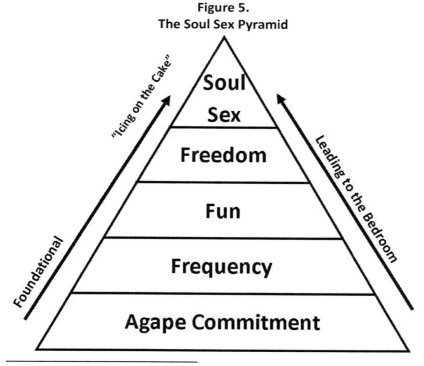

---

[81] Philippians 2:3-4 says "...in humility consider others better than yourselves. Each of you should look not only to your own interests, but also to the interests of others." Jesus should be our model (see verses 5-8).

You Need a Process

What you need is a way to move you as a couple together up the pyramid—a process that shows husbands how to lead sexually and that show wives how to follow. It's going to take some knowledge, which this book will provide, and some communication and commitment, which you *both* must provide. A husband learning to lovingly lead his wife to greater sexual intimacy (and a wife learning to follow) is a process—you grow into it.

The Dilemma

The main problem lies in how married couples tend to relate to each other about sex. In every other area of marriage, we know that we must grow into married oneness from singleness.

Think about it—you know that you have to adjust and stretch to care for another person, to learn to be considerate, to blend your unique viewpoints on finances into a productive whole, and to make a thousand other compromises and collaborations on diverse life decisions—from the proverbial question of where to squeeze the toothpaste to the all-important issue of how to discipline children.

Some of these steps toward oneness have simple solutions (get two tubes of toothpaste); others may come with much "weeping and gnashing of teeth." But by and large, we know that resolution comes down to good communication. We must understand each other, work it out, play by fair rules, forgive often—and our marriage ends up the better for it.

However, when it comes to sex, the rules seem to change. Although it's the most powerful tool God has given married couples to promote oneness, in most marriages, sex is the most awkward, least-discussed topic of conversation. Whether it's going well or not so well, couples often remain silent about it with each other.

Why don't we know that great sex requires great communication, and that we need God in the equation? Most couples' silence and lack of growth in sexual intimacy can be traced back to our nemesis, the Devil.

Ultimately, Satan is behind every strategy to keep husband and wife from experiencing the oneness God created. We surveyed some of his many strategies in Chapter One, but generally, he works through the world and tripping up our flesh.

The world system teaches the enemy's lies and discouragement about one of God's greatest gifts from our earliest days. The fallenness of our flesh produces men who are reluctant to lead because of lack of confidence and women who are hindered in their sexual expression by past wounds from abuse or words, which lead to insecurity.

Here is a typical scenario that the LEAD process is designed to help. A wife has some wound or issue that makes her:

1) inhibited and timid

2) feel unattractive and less than sexy at times (though her husband thinks she is beautiful).

When you add these two factors to the regular busyness of a full life, exhaustion from kids, and the fact that she probably has a naturally lower sex drive than her husband, you have a recipe for a marriage that is lacking in soul sex.

The wife's wounds work to greatly reduce the comfort she has with a very strong desire in her husband: soul-stirring sexual intimacy, fantasies a man has of erotic, free, passionate, loud, experimental, unique kinds of sex as well as a more flirtatious and romantic everyday non-sexual relationship (words, notes, flirts) that build desire and anticipation for soul sex. (It is not uncommon in good, solid Christian marriages for a husband to feel that he and his wife have sex one-third to one-half as much as he desires.)

The husband has his own wounds and weaknesses as well. Just as Adam was silent in the Garden when the stakes were high, so men today often forfeit leadership in their intimate life. Sadly, most couples end up settling for the lowest common denominator in their sex life instead of the greatest level of intimacy possible.

The Lowest Common Denominator

The lowest common denominator (LCD) is when you settle on an intimacy level somewhat less than soul sex (in frequency, fun, freedom, passion, or all of these). The decision is made almost subconsciously, in an effort to avoid rocking the boat and any uncomfortable discussion (see Figure 6). Perhaps neither partner is fully satisfied with their intimate life, but neither is dissatisfied enough to get to the tipping point of change. Or, one or both of you is

LCD – neither partner is fully satisfied, but neither is dissatisfied enough to get to the tipping point of change.

dissatisfied enough, but does not know how to go about the awkward task of increasing your intimacy.

Maybe you've even talked and agreed to work on the gap you have in expectations, but you tend to fall back to the LCD. You have sex regularly (but not quite frequently enough for one of you). Your wife may be insecure about wearing lingerie, your husband may not be as tender and mood-

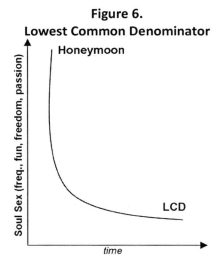

Figure 6.
Lowest Common Denominator

setting as intimacy requires, or your erotic life tends toward familiar, tamer encounters. There's nothing wrong with the intimacy you do share—it's just the lowest common denominator.

The danger is more than just simply missing the icing on the cake. The LCD represents a lack of intimacy fulfillment for one or both partners. This leads to disappointment, which if not dealt with, can lead to resentment. Resentment is the enemy of the oneness God meant for you to have (see Figure 7).

But there is a better way.

Figure 7.
Where the Lowest Common Denominator Leads

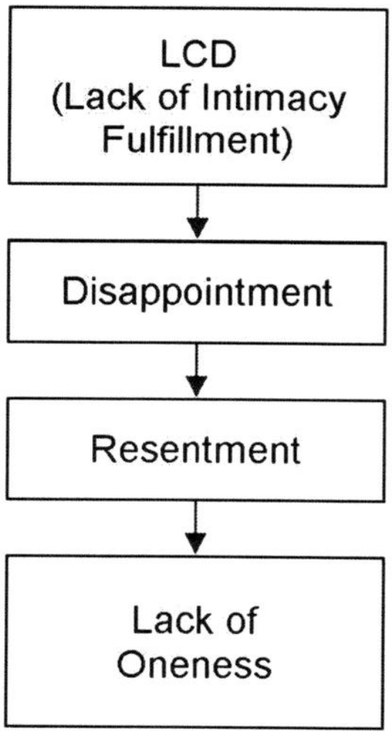

```
        ┌─────────────────────┐
        │         LCD         │
        │ (Lack of Intimacy   │
        │    Fulfillment)     │
        └─────────────────────┘
                   │
                   ▼
        ┌─────────────────────┐
        │   Disappointment    │
        └─────────────────────┘
                   │
                   ▼
        ┌─────────────────────┐
        │     Resentment      │
        └─────────────────────┘
                   │
                   ▼
        ┌─────────────────────┐
        │      Lack of        │
        │      Oneness        │
        └─────────────────────┘
```

Does this Sound Familiar?

There is a spiritual process that flows directly out of the gospel that couples can employ in order to see God restore the gift He intended for them. This chapter is the explanation of that process. But first, consider men's possible reactions.

Unmet and unresolved sexual expectations[82] tend to create the lowest common denominator of intimacy within a couple. How? Without a process to work through the expectations, you land at the lowest level of intimacy you both want to experience.

This results in disappointment (especially on the part of the man). The thief has succeeded in stealing the joy God meant for you to have in bringing you together.

What a man does next is the key to whether he stays disappointed or he fights together with his wife to get back what the enemy has taken.

Fight or Flight

Without insight about what's going on or the tools to work through their expectations, men often do one of two things: they get angry or they go passive, like Adam.

It looks like this (see Figure 8). A man's wife is not meeting his expectations in frequency, freedom, fun, or passion; as a couple, they've settled on some lowest common denominator. He is disappointed, hurt, and frustrated.

He lashes out in anger, either demanding to get his way or withdrawing with a bad attitude. There may be a whole cycle of anger leading to consequences in the relationship. Of course, his wife feels the resentment, but she may not understand it. The end result is that there is a lack of oneness in the relationship.

Or, actually much more common than getting angry, a man can go passive when faced with the disappointment of unmet expectations. Perhaps he doesn't even let his desires be known because he's asked before and felt rejected. This can be anything from simply backing down at the critical moments that could increase intimacy to a whole cycle of not stepping up to lead in the relationship.

---

[82] We'll talk much more about expectations in Chapter Four.

In this case, the husband feels resentment toward his wife because of his frustration and disappointment. The final result here again is a lack of oneness. By the way, we're picking on men, but when women's expectations are unmet, they can also get angry or go passive.

But I will show you a more excellent way...

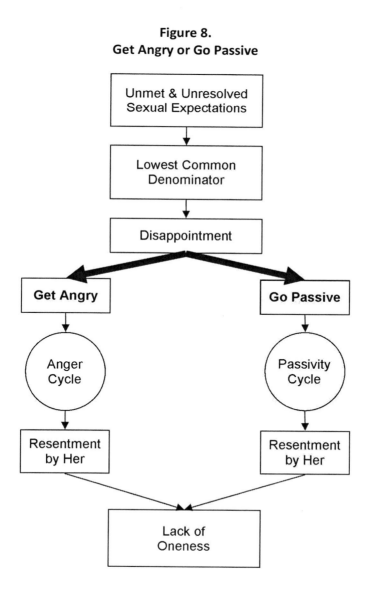

Figure 8.
Get Angry or Go Passive

It Doesn't Have to Be this Way!

What if we could break the cycle? Disappointment is inevitable. (We are fallen people in a fallen world under attack by Satan). But, what if, instead of getting angry or going passive, there was a third option with better results.

Imagine that you both felt the freedom to try something totally new or different (and passionate)? And the stakes were low because if this particular sex experiment doesn't work out, then either of you have the freedom to wake the other up in a couple of hours and be pleased the way he or she normally likes *on the same day*!

If that sounds like an unbelievable dream fantasy, then you need the LEAD process to find out why that seems so unreachable. If soul sex is as important to oneness as Scripture suggests, making it a serious goal of our marriage is effort well invested. I love what Pastor Mark Driscoll says about it: "You're not that tired!"[83]

Throughout your marriage, you have grown in the area of finances, parenting, decision-making—now it's time to learn to lead (and follow) in intimacy.

Be a Servant—by Leading

In John 13, Jesus gave us the perfect picture of godly servant leadership when He washed Peter's feet. The scene has much to teach us about the way husbands should lead wives.

First, notice that Jesus was confident in His authority, and that confidence allowed Him to humble Himself and lead.

3 Jesus knew that the Father had put all things under his power, and that he had come from God and was returning to God;

---

[83] Driscoll. "The Peasant Princess: Let Him Kiss Me.", September 21, 2008.

4 so he got up from the meal, took off his outer clothing, and wrapped a towel around his waist.[84]

Husband, are you a little uncomfortable with the comparison of you to Jesus? You shouldn't be. Ephesians 5:23 says,

For the husband is the head [leader] of the wife as Christ is the head of the church.

Who decided that? God. The issue of husbandly leadership has nothing to do with who's smarter—or even who is more spiritually mature. It is based on God giving authority to the husband to lead the marriage.

If you accept your God-given role as Jesus did, humbly and with the motive to serve God and not yourself, then you can be completely confident in leading your wife. You are not acting from a selfish motive, but from a godly one.

Perhaps you have hurt or bitterness. Don't miss that Jesus is about to wash Judas Iscariot's feet,[85] the man Jesus knows will betray Him in a few hours. When your love and leadership flow from God, there is an endless supply for whatever the need, no matter how great.

Don't try to lead until you have settled the issue of where your authority comes from. Verses 3-4 say that Jesus knew He had authority from God, *so* He was able to serve. We must do the same.

Next, notice that Jesus was a selfless servant for His disciples' good:

5 After that, he poured water into a basin and began to wash his disciples' feet, drying them with the towel that was wrapped around him.

---

[84] John 13:3-4.
[85] See John 13:2.

Dirty feet were a nuisance at the dinner table,[86] and the job of washing them generally went to a paid servant. In the absence of a servant, it went to the person of lowest social standing, certainly not the host or rabbi.

Jesus took up the basin and towel and turned humanity's view of greatness upside down. Just as Jesus humbly served those who follow Him, a husband is called to be a servant for his wife's good, putting her needs above his own.[87]

Of utmost importance for husbands to grasp, however, is that Jesus was a servant-*leader* to Peter. He knew what was best for Peter even if Peter himself didn't, and He didn't let Peter sway Him from what was best.

> *6 He came to Simon Peter, who said to him, "Lord, are you going to wash my feet?"*
> *7 Jesus replied, "You do not realize now what I am doing, but later you will understand."*
> *8 "No," said Peter, "you shall never wash my feet." Jesus answered, "Unless I wash you, you have no part with me."*
> *9 "Then, Lord," Simon Peter replied, "not just my feet but my hands and my head as well!"*
> *10 Jesus answered, "A person who has had a bath needs only to wash his feet; his whole body is clean. And you are clean, though not every one of you."*

Jesus was teaching Peter and the disciples that to have a relationship with Christ (symbolized by the meal together) meant that we would have to allow Him to

---

[86] Hot climate, open sandals, and donkey as the primary mode of transportation along the same streets people walk on—perhaps we should say dirty feet were a *major* nuisance at the dinner table, which was low to the ground.

[87] Philippians 2:3-8.

cleanse us from the daily sin we're susceptible to. Our whole body doesn't have to be washed again (we're still saved), but to have close fellowship with the Lord, we need Him to continually take away the stain of our daily brushes with sin.

As Peter's *leader*, Jesus was insistent on doing for him what He knew was right and what Peter needed (washing his feet only, not his whole body), even if Peter didn't grasp it himself yet.

Husband, that's what God is calling you to do with your wife: lead her into something that will be good for you both. God wants you to use the leadership role He's given you in His power and for His purpose to selflessly serve your wife by leading her.

Bill Lawrence sums up Christ's example for us this way:

> This is servant leadership: doing what God wants at all costs, even at the price of resistance and confrontation from those we serve by leading. One of the ways we function as servant leaders is when we go against the will of others in order to accomplish God's will in their lives.[88]

Everything Jesus did was for Peter's good, though it wasn't what Peter wanted at first. Jesus' motives weren't selfish at all. When your motives are right (from God), you as a husband can confidently lead because you know God placed you in authority. Servant leaders serve their wives by leading their marriage to God's design.

What Servant Leadership is NOT

The biblical concept of servant leadership is NOT a license to be selfish, bullying, lazy, or abusive. In fact, it's the exact opposite! Husbands, do not misinterpret the definition above as a way to mistreat your wife. Our

---

[88] Bill Lawrence, *Effective Pastoring* (Nashville: Word Publishing, 1999), 94.

model is Christ putting His disciples' needs above His own. Just to be clear, you should NEVER force or compel your mate into something sexually she is not comfortable with.

Until you're ready to lead like Jesus (humbly, lovingly serving *and* leading out of God-given authority), you'll come up short in leading your marriage to greater intimacy. Men, take some time to consider John 13 and ask God to make you a godly servant leader in your marriage.

Ladies, you would do well to also consider John 13, and ask God to help you be receptive to godly servant leadership. Your marriage growing in intimacy and oneness depends on it.

The LEAD Process

The attitude and approach of servant leadership is vital to achieving success in growing in intimacy. Remember, our goal is to tear down any divisive wall between you and build up a protective wall around your marriage. It's also to experience soul sex, everything God intended in His original design for sex in marriage, before the enemy came at the Fall to steal, kill, and destroy everything God had made for His highest creation to enjoy.

To achieve these worthy goals, you have to get beyond getting angry or going passive. Thank God, there is a third option with much greater results. Instead, you can lead to the bedroom. In fact, we affectionately call the process to achieve these goals *Leading to the Bedroom* (or the LEAD Process, for short).

Leading to the Bedroom is a four-step servant leadership (and servant-following) process with relational, spiritual, action, and progress-oriented tools for a husband to lead his wife to greater sexual intimacy. It involves self-reflection as well as communication with your spouse.

We're going to examine each step of the LEAD process in detail in the coming chapters, but here is an overview (see Figures 9 and 10):

L – Learn about Your Mate

Learn about Your Mate is a planned process of humble communication with your spouse for the purpose of understanding your mate's desires and needs so that you can move together toward greater intimacy. It actually involves two phases, Prayer and Discovery.

Prayer gets you focused on God and His desires for your intimacy. Discovery is carried out with the spirit of Matthew 7:5: "...first take the plank out of your own eye, and then you will see clearly to remove the speck from your brother's eye."

The primary tool for *Learning about your Mate* is a Learning Talk.

E – Experience the Gospel

Experience the Gospel brings God's good news to bear on your intimate life. Wife, what if you've conditioned your husband not to pursue because when he made the effort, you didn't reward him—the very thing you desire most, you've taught him not to do. Do you see how Satan has stolen from you both?

What would it look like if you not only said yes, but you invited (made it easy/fun) your husband to pursue you. This happens when you stop believing the lies of the enemy and start trusting God's good news for your intimacy.

Figure 9.
LEAD – A Better Way

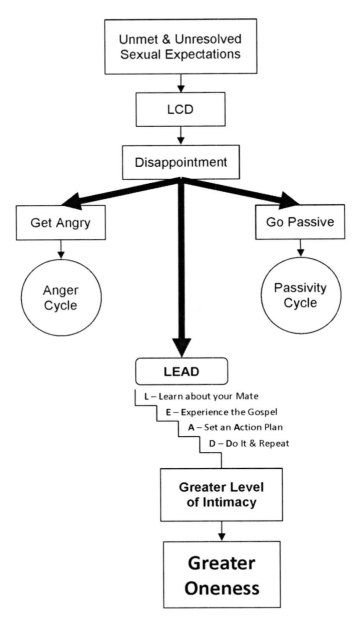

Figure 10.
The LEAD Process

L Learn about your Mate
Prayer & Discovery
Pray, Share, Understand
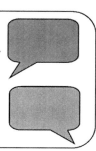

E Experience the Gospel
Repent & Believe
Repent, Believe, Walk

A Set an Action Plan
Commit to
Hot Pursuit
Frequency, Fun, Freedom

D Do it and Repeat
Follow-Through
& Progress
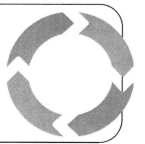

Husband, you're likely also believing some lies that hinder you from experiencing God's design. You'll identify and repent of them in this step, too. Then you can trust God for His good news.

Your primary tools are Repent & Believe Worksheets to help you identify Satan's lies that you have fallen for and God's truths that you can trust.

A – Set an Action Plan

Your new beliefs won't transform your intimacy unless you put them into action. James said, "faith without works is dead."[89]

Husband, what would it look like if you became a romantic surprise-springer, gift-giver, date-planner, and hand holder?

Wife, what if your husband never had to suffer through the "awkward ask" again because your first answer was yes?

These are just a couple of the key areas you'll learn to set progressive goals in to lead your marriage to its full intimate potential.

Your primary tool in *Set an Action Plan* is an Intimacy Action Plan for your marriage based on the soul sex pyramid. This is a custom plan you will develop together by agreeing on goals that you put on your calendar.

D – Do it and Evaluate

Let's face it: what gets measured gets done. But because sex is such an emotional, intimate topic, we don't measure how we're doing in this area. In the area of personal finances, Dave Ramsey has turned the world

---

[89] James 2:17.

upside down with his Baby Steps,[90] which if followed will make you financially successful. But we haven't had any Baby Steps for our sexual intimacy—until now.

Following the intimacy action plan you developed in Step 3 of the LEAD Process, you will now *Do It and Repeat*. This means you'll actually carry out some or all of your action plan and then start the process over, taking advantage in this next iteration of the progress made in the last. You'll again:

Learn from Your Mate. You'll evaluate how everything is going—what's awesome and what still needs work.

Experience the Gospel. In light of your new plateau of sexual intimacy, what lies have surfaced that need to be repented of? What new aspect of God's truth do you need to trust in?

Set an Action Plan. Armed with your new insight, you'll set an action plan based on where you are now and where you want to go.

Do It and Repeat. This is a cyclical process where after each action plan, you use the LEAD process again to evaluate your progress and fine-tune your future growth in intimacy.

Your primary tools to *Do It and Repeat* are LEAD graphs, which show the next plateau you want to achieve and a timeline for how quickly you want to get there.

Each of these steps is vitally important in the process. In Chapters Four through Seven, we'll look at each step in detail.

From Plateau to Plateau

Wherever you are now in your intimacy (unless you're just getting back from your honeymoon) is a plateau

---

[90] If you haven't yet joined the Financial Peace revolution, check out www.DaveRamsey.com.

you're on...even if it's a good plateau, is it the greatest level of intimacy possible?

If you've been stuck in a less-than-satisfying plateau for a while, the prospect of LEADing to greater sexual intimacy may seem overwhelming. Don't listen to lies from the enemy, who would love to discourage you.

Rather, remember how to eat an elephant—one bite at a time. The LEAD process helps you move from plateau to plateau in incremental steps. What bite-sized progress do you agree to make together in a one or two month timeframe? You decide together in steps L, E, and A, and then carry out your plan in step D. At the end, you've reached a higher and more satisfying plateau, a level closer to the oneness the Creator designed for your marriage. Then, you repeat the process to reach an even higher plateau. It looks like Figure 11.

Figure 11.
LEADing from Plateau to Plateau

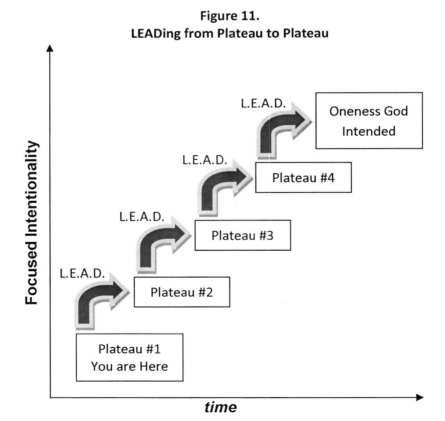

We'll come back to this graph more and define your specific plateau in Chapter Six, *Set an Action Plan*, but for now, just recognize that you'll make progress incrementally.

Some Practical Pointers

As with every skill you learn, you may not be great at it at first, but if you give up early on, you'll never get good at it. Here's some practical advice from our experience using the LEAD process to grow to greater intimacy.

Proceed with caution. As you start, you both need to realize that this is an incredibly vulnerable process.

The road of male leadership is fraught with pitfalls. A man takes a huge risk when he makes a clear, vulnerable, real, and true step toward asking his wife to come with him to a deeper place of soul intimacy in satisfying deep strong desires he has.

If this request fades into the noise of busyness, work, raising kids—i.e. life, it will be much harder to make progress in the future. Wife, after such a heart-baring plea has failed, it will be much harder for him to risk leading in intimacy again. Don't miss your opportunity to affirm your husband for stepping up to lead by whole-heartedly following his leadership.

A wife's path to greater sexual intimacy is not without its perils either. It can be very intimidating for a woman when her husband is transparent about his desires. The danger for her is personal: it may make her feel defensive to find he is not content with the intimate life they already share.

Discouragement can set in, wondering whether she'll ever be able to please her husband. "I already do more sensual sex acts than I'm really comfortable with," she may think from her perspective of timidity and insecurity. Husband, tread carefully and caringly, treating your wife as a daughter of the King.

Affirm each other! Because this is a treacherous path, take every opportunity to affirm each other. Tell your spouse often how much you love him or her and that you are together on this journey. Wife, praise his adventurous heart and be thankful that he has a desire to explore your sexuality together. Husband, affirm her beauty and sensuality and be grateful for her willingness to follow.

This entire process should be encouraging and not guilt-ridden. Do not use the LEAD concepts as a weapon against each other. If discussing your sexual intimacy drives a wedge between you, you have missed the whole point of sexual intimacy being about oneness. That's not to say there won't be some periods of stretching as you realize false beliefs you need to shed.

No buts! In the preface, we say that we now talk more freely as a couple about intimacy, we have increased our frequency, and we've made sex more fun, erotic, and pleasing to both of us. But be assured that did not happen overnight. It took *two years* of intentional and systematic focus on LEADing to the Bedroom.

You may be tempted to read of our success and come up with all the "buts":

But, you may say, we were more mature than you are.
But I must be a better leader.
But my wife is a better follower.
But, but, but...

No buts—we worked at the process, and we had ups and downs and some awkward disappointments along the way.

But we will tell you this—we would not trade where we are now for ANYTHING in the world. Our relationship is warmer (hotter, really) and better in every way. Don't make excuses, and don't give up!

Play to your team strengths. As you start to LEAD, take advantage of the strengths each of you have. If one of you is a planner, don't make fun of that person—rather enjoy the security of plans. If one is carefree, work that into the beauty of your intimacy together.

Don't treat the process lightly. Don't forget that the enemy is actively working to keep you from LEADing. We've put a lot of thought (not to mention personal trial and error) into how to make progress. If you stop every time you hit a hard season, guess what—the enemy will make sure you hit a hard season.

We recommend you do the process just as we've outlined it for six months so the enemy doesn't steal your time through busyness. When we tell you to do a learning talk once a month (defined in the next chapter), write it on the calendar. When you stick to the schedule, the intervals are short enough to course correct if necessary without getting far off track. Each of the steps, L, E, A, and D, should initially be about one- or two-month segments—one month if you don't have kids, two months if you do.

Take bite-sized chunks. For most couples, you're making great progress if you:

L: Have one learning talk per month.

E: Turn from two lies you've believed and trust in God's truth. You should only move on to tackle more lies once you both feel you've achieved success. (You may battle one pervasive lie on an ongoing basis.)

A: Actively work on two action steps per month (i.e., increase frequency and get rid of the awkward ask (as opposed to these *plus* experiment with more erotic lovemaking)).

D: Commit to one month (two if you have kids) of doing your current action plan, and then have your next learning talk, taking advantage of this month's progress.

Don't fail to do the LEAD process because you hit a challenge. That's how the enemy wants to keep stealing from you. Hang in there, because the payoff is worth it!

Burn the Ships, and All In!

Legend has it that Spanish conquistador Hernando Cortez burned his ships upon arrival to the New World so that his 600 men wouldn't be tempted to turn back from the challenge ahead. By removing retreat as an option, he and his men were forced to forge ahead. That's commitment to the cause!

Today, husband and wife, is D-Day for you, Decision Day, when you decide that there is a better way—that the greatest gift for joy and the greatest catalyst for greater oneness will no longer be wasted on your marriage because of fallenness.

We must tell you, if you want more frequent, fun, free and passionate sex and all the benefits it brings to your relationship, it will take a serious commitment by both partners. In fact, if either of you are a little half-hearted in your commitment, let me warn you that beginning this process and stopping short can actually drive you further apart, as one partner's hopes are let down by the other.

So, as you read and understand the process of LEADing to the Bedroom, both of you must fully commit to the process in order to realize the fruit that God intends in your relationship.

There is a term in Poker for when you lay all your chips on the table and make the bet of your life; you're "all in!" From here on out, in order to increase intimacy, both of you need to be "all in"...oh wait, you already promised that the day you got married, right? Before you turn the page, reaffirm to your spouse that you are "all in!"

Get ready to LEAD to the Bedroom.

A Wife's Take

Ladies, letting your husband lead in this area can be a bit scary. It really boils down to this: Do you really want to have oneness in your marriage, or do you just say you want it?

If you're just saying it, then you're not willing to do the work it requires. There will always be something else that takes precedence over a great sex life and a fulfilled husband: kids, work, friends, ministry, or God forbid, even a favorite TV show!

Girls, you have an opportunity here. Believe me, your husband will be interested in this marriage book more than any other because it promises more fun and frequent sex. Dave and I have agonized throughout planning this book about how to get *women* to want to participate in the process.

Your husband's needs are more than merely sexual. He really needs to know that you are there for him; sex is a very tangible way to show that. Ephesians 5 affirms that his *greatest* need from you is respect. God calls us to respect our husbands and follow their lead. When he has the guts to say, "Arise and come with me," you will honor God and bless your guy when you say, "Here I come."

When Satan stole our "unashamed-ness" in the Garden, he stole the intimacy we and our husbands desperately want. Fight, together with your husband, to take it back. I know you want to have a marriage that's more fulfilling than you've even dared to dream of—the way God designed it. I'm praying that you won't trade it for lesser things.

Chapter Four
L – Learn About Your Mate
Prayer & Discovery

And let us consider how we may spur one another on toward love and good deeds.
—Hebrews 10:24

When you're not speaking to each other, you can be sure the enemy is speaking to both of you.
—Dave Jones

A problem well-defined is a problem half-solved.
—John Dewey

Once God showed me I wasn't leading my wife in the area of intimacy, I whole-heartedly committed to start. But that was only half the battle. I would lead, but how willing and able would my shy, insecure wife be to follow me on this journey?

Still separated by an ocean at that point, I wrote her the most carefully worded email of my life, wanting to share this powerful leading from God without spooking her. Her response was beautiful: "I trust you, and I will follow you; you know my insecurities." We were already headed down the path toward greater intimacy.

As soon as I returned, I took her to our favorite bed & breakfast. There, on a walk in the woods, I poured out my heart. As the conversation turned more intimate, we found a bench in the woods (how thoughtful of God!). Through unashamed communication, we understood more about each other and our intimacy that day in two hours than we had in the first thirteen years of our marriage. This was our first learning talk regarding our sexual intimacy.

Define the (Sexual) Relationship

When a couple is dating, one of the hardest and most significant discussions they will have is the "DTR," (define the relationship). I had my DTR with Katie on our first date. You could say I was eager...it was love at first sight.

The purpose of this all-important conversation is for a guy to let a girl he's dating know what he, as the leader, thinks about their relationship—to clarify where he is on the scale from "just friends" to "let's set a wedding date."

With a DTR, a girl doesn't have to guess at a guy's motives, risking her heart in the process. Because matters of the heart take courage and vulnerability, many a guy has been content to keep dating without any talk of commitment.

After marriage, the need for courage and vulnerability grows, not lessens. Sexual intimacy can be an extremely difficult subject to talk about with your mate because our enemy has so thoroughly attempted to steal the blessing of sex in marriage. Men, if you want a better sex life, you need to talk to your wives. You need to have the DT(S)R. Don't worry; we'll coach you through it.

We Don't Talk about Sex

It's a fact: we don't really discuss sex in our culture. We see plenty of it in the movies, on TV, and on the internet, but none of that expresses God's design for sex as the greatest catalyst for oneness in marriage.

And we're not talking about it in church or at home. Most of the men I know say their dads never really talked with them about sex—and those who did generally didn't approach it from a spiritual perspective.

In fact, Dr. Douglas Weiss says over 95 percent of men's talks with their fathers about sex lasted fewer than three minutes.[91] Mine lasted less than one minute on a fishing trip at age thirteen. It went something like this:

> **Dad**: "Your mom said I should talk to you about sex. Grandpa didn't tell me anything. Do you have any questions?"
> **Me:** "No."
> **Dad**: (long silence with internal sigh of relief[92]) Getting any bites?

In the absence of father-to-son instruction, Weiss says fourteen to sixteen-year-old boys usually learn about sex from other fourteen to sixteen-year-old boys.[93] Talk about the blind leading the blind! I remember my friend in eighth grade enlightening me with the knowledge that "the snake goes up your wife"—call me naïve, but I didn't know what "the snake" was or where specifically it was supposed to go, but I do remember the distinct feeling that this was something I shouldn't be talking about. This friend also showed me a picture of a naked woman from *Playboy*, which he cut to carry in his wallet. Our culture is sex-crazed but truth-starved.

Unfortunately, couples tend to carry this lack of talking about intimacy into marriage, especially as misunderstandings come up. The enemy so thoroughly attaches shame and insecurity to sex that husbands and wives often shy away from talking openly about it. While they desperately crave true intimacy, they often can't

---

[91] Weiss, *Sex, Men & God*, xii.
[92] I included this not to poke fun at my dad but as an example of the enemy's successful strategy to keep men from the truth in this area.
[93] Weiss, *Sex, Men & God*, xii.

bring themselves to communicate it to the one person God gave them to meet that desire.

This is our major problem: great sex starts with communication, but our churches and parents didn't talk to us about sex, our friends gave us useless information about sex, husbands and wives don't talk to each other about sex, and we don't talk to God about sex.

Great sex starts with communication, but we don't talk about sex.

Learning about your mate, the first step in LEADing to the bedroom, will help you change that. Don't worry; we're going to take it slow. If you commit to LEADing, you will have *many* learning talks throughout your marriage. They'll get easier; you'll enjoy them more as you go; and you'll go deeper in understanding each other.

So, when is the last time you defined your sexual relationship with your wife? I mean, had a really good talk after which you both walked away understanding each other? Even more importantly, when is the last time you prayed about your sex life?

In this chapter, you're going to learn how to ask God to increase your intimacy with your spouse (learning from Him), as well as how to have a great *real* conversation with your spouse about your intimacy. Learning about your mate has a vertical (prayer) and a horizontal (discovery) component.

PRAYER

By praying before you have this intimate conversation with so much at stake, you recognize God's place and yours.

Husband, you are acknowledging your humility and dependence on the Lord to wholeheartedly lead your wife in this sensitive area.

Wife, you are acknowledging your humility and dependence on the Lord to submit to your husband and participate fully in the process of becoming closer through sexual intimacy.

No matter what obstacles you've faced in the past, you are now asking the God of the universe to bring His wisdom and power to bear on your marital intimacy.

Learning from God does several great things for you. It helps you clarify (and purify) your motives. Knowing you've asked God's help allows you to let your guard down. You're asking Him to lead you and to make learning about your mate a successful step toward oneness in your marriage.

What specifically should you pray to prepare for your learning talk with your spouse? Initially, you may want to pray the following husband's and wife's prayer. As you repeat the process, you will have more issues specific to your relationship to pray about.

Husband's Learning Prayer

Lord, I'm seeking You for how to lovingly LEAD my beautiful bride to trust me without fear. Please forgive me for any ways that I have been a barrier to greater oneness. Help me to be selfless as I grow in this area. Give me Your power to be a godly leader. Help me know how to lead her. Lord, please heal her from any wounds she has, and please use me in the healing process. Please, by Jesus' work in us, give us a full, abundant soul oneness that You intend for us, but that the thief has tried to steal. I'm trusting You to do something GREAT in our marriage. I ask this in Jesus' name. Amen.

Wife's Learning Prayer

Lord, I'm seeking You for how to respectfully follow my husband's leadership as he seeks to lead us to greater intimacy. Please forgive me for any ways that I have been a barrier to greater oneness. Help me to be selfless as I grow in this area. Give me Your power to be a godly wife. Help me know how to draw close to my husband. Lord, please heal him from any wounds he has, and please use me in the healing process. Help me encourage him to be a bold and loving leader. Please, by Jesus' work in us, give us a full, abundant soul oneness that the thief tried to steal. I'm trusting You to do something GREAT in our marriage. I ask this in Jesus' name. Amen.

After praying, sit still for a few minutes and let God speak to you. Keep a journal and write down anything God impresses on you. You've talked to God; expect Him to respond back to you. Read a devotional. If you don't yet read your Bible every day (or listen to it on mp3), this would be a great time to start this spiritual discipline—it is the best way to learn from God. (Also, listening to great preaching on demand for free on iTunes podcasts is an awesome privilege granted only in this generation. Take advantage of it.)

To the Husband

One of the best ways to increase intimacy with your wife is to pray with her.

Husband, you can and should be praying about greater oneness by yourself on a regular basis, but there's an even better way! Since this whole process is about increasing intimacy with your wife, I'm going to let you in on a great secret. One of the best ways to increase intimacy with your wife is to pray *with* her!

Since you are the leader, you need to initiate this. Let me warn you: it is difficult. Pastor Andy Stanley shared with a group of pastors once that every man he knows (including himself) finds it hard to initiate praying with his wife—but Andy shared that when he does, it brings closeness like nothing else. I have found this to be absolutely true in my marriage. I think it's difficult because our enemy is trying to steal our oneness.[94]

DISCOVERY

After praying, you are ready to focus on the horizontal component of learning, the process of discovery through open discussion with your spouse. First things first—you must come to a basic agreement together, a truce if you will. The agreement is this: it is good to talk about sex. If you in any way make your partner feel ashamed about opening up to you about sex, you cannot grow in oneness.

Let's call a truce: It is good to talk about sex.

This topic is very intimate and possibly uncomfortable, so it is vital to set the stage and choose the timing carefully for this critical talk or series of talks.

The stakes for this discussion with your spouse are very high. The enemy would love nothing more than to take what is potentially the most powerful step toward oneness you've ever taken and turn it into a divisive wedge, damaging the very oneness you're working toward.

Gear Up

But you can set yourselves up for success by being prepared spiritually against the inevitable attack of the enemy. He doesn't want you and your spouse to win at intimacy. But Paul told us how to gear up for victory. I wouldn't have a learning talk without suiting up. Consider Paul's instructions for battle in Ephesians chapter six:

---

[94] Andy Stanley also pondered why it is so difficult to pray with our wives. He hypothesized that it is our male pride, as praying makes us very vulnerable with our wives. The Holy Spirit in you can defeat pride and the enemy's attack.

10 Finally, be strong in the Lord and in his mighty power.

God's power will help you win the battle against the enemy.

11 Put on the full armor of God so that you can take your stand against the devil's schemes.

Want to win against the enemy's tactics? Put on God's armor. Don't go to battle naked. (Save that for encounters with your beloved!)

12 For our struggle is not against flesh and blood, but against the rulers, against the authorities, against the powers of this dark world and against the spiritual forces of evil in the heavenly realms.

Your spouse is not your enemy. It's Satan we must fight against. You and your spouse are on the same team. Don't give any impression otherwise.

13 Therefore put on the full armor of God, so that when the day of evil comes, you may be able to stand your ground, and after you have done everything, to stand.

God's armor helps you stand up under the pressure when the enemy attacks your relationship.

14 Stand firm then, with the belt of truth buckled around your waist,

What's the real truth here? We're on the same team. We're committed to each other. We're working toward oneness. God has provided sexual intimacy to catalyze greater oneness in our marriage. Don't believe lies that say otherwise. Keep truth close by, close as your belt.

with the breastplate of righteousness in place,

Christ has made me righteous through His sacrifice. I can have the confidence to lead (or follow) because He has made me righteous. Thank God His righteousness protects me, and not my own!

15 and with your feet fitted with the readiness that comes from the gospel of peace.[95]

I am ready to lead and/or follow because of the good news that we can trust Him.

16 In addition to all this, take up the shield of faith, with which you can extinguish all the flaming arrows of the evil one.

Believing (faith) that God has made me righteous and that God can help me lead (or follow) keeps me protected against the enemy's lies to the contrary.

17 Take the helmet of salvation and the sword of the Spirit, which is the word of God.

Lord, protect my mind, reminding me that you have saved me and will deliver us to greater intimacy. Help me use the truth of God's Word to combat lies.

18 And pray in the Spirit on all occasions with all kinds of prayers and requests. With this in mind, be alert and always keep on praying for all the saints.

---

[95] We'll examine the gospel in greater detail in the next chapter.

Don't forget that the greatest weapon is asking God to fight this spiritual battle.

Setting

In addition to preparing for the learning talk spiritually, setting the mood well will stack the deck in your favor.

You should have this talk at a time and in a setting when you normally have your best talks. You should schedule your learning talk for an occasion when you won't be rushed and when the kids are taken care of. A state away from them is best! (I'm only half kidding.)

Katie and I have our best talks primarily in three places. She loves bed-and-breakfasts—after a lovely breakfast we have often talked the day away about the most intimate of subjects while enjoying a beautiful, private setting.

But don't think that these talks require that you spend lots of money. We have also had great talks at restaurants. A romantic dinner or even a quiet breakfast place with atmosphere come to mind as places that we have connected. Obviously, some things may be harder to share with wait staff bound to show up at any time and other patrons nearby. We often start a planned talk at dinner and then continue it in the car.

Actually, on a car trip is one of the best times to have an intimate talk. Neither of you has to look the other in the eye, which can be helpful if you're expressing your feelings or desires in ways you never have before. Also, you don't have to respond right away—there is plenty of time to think about what you're feeling without the other person wondering why you aren't responding immediately.

Katie and I joke that long car trips are dangerous for us. Almost every major decision we've ever made (buying our first house, going to seminary, where to invest, and when to have children) happened when we were on a long car ride and had time to talk and dream together.

Since these have proven to be relaxing, non-threatening, conversation-inducing settings for us, I like to schedule a learning talk trifecta: nice dinner, bed-and-breakfast stay and a car ride there and back. Add a thoughtful gift and if you've prayed and put on God's armor beforehand, you almost can't lose at having a positive intimate conversation.

The difference between a great learning talk that results in greater sexual intimacy and a lousy one that sets you back is preparation—spiritual and practical. Don't have a learning talk if you haven't prepared.

Certainly, none of us has enough money to have the super-date weekend described above too often. But there are countless other ways to set up for a great learning talk, and you need to find what works for you as a couple.

Taking care of the kids, doing dishes and laundry, taking the trash out without being asked, and preparing a bath for my wife while I do these household chores can also create the right setting.

My point is simply that you must think about these elements. Never underestimate the importance of timing and setting in leading to the bedroom.

Husband, I encourage you to take a moment right now to get a date on the calendar for your first learning talk and write down a few ideas for location, atmosphere, and setting.

Date for Learning Talk: _____

Setting Plans: _____

_____

_____

_____

Three Goals of Learning Discovery

You've set the stage for a win! Now, what exactly is a learning talk? It is a regular periodic conversation with your spouse for the purpose of casting vision, unearthing buried expectations, and communicating clearly about your sex life.

A learning talk is a regular periodic conversation to cast vision, unearth expectations, and communicate clearly about sex.

Learning talks follow Solomon's and his bride's example in Scripture.[96] While couples today often don't communicate what they really want from each other, Solomon and his bride spent eight chapters— stretching from courtship to old age—talking about sex!

What's your vision for your sex life? It can be as simple as "I want sex more often" or "I want to take the next step in more adventurous intimacy." Casting vision is simply painting a picture (something the other person can grasp) of the values you share for greater oneness.

What expectations do you have? For the ones that are being met, do you give praise and appreciation? For the ones that aren't, are you honest with your spouse about the fact that you have them? Are you able to share expectations in a healthy, productive way, or do your attempts at intimate conversation become a barrier to intimacy?

How are you at communicating about sex? Does your spouse "get" you? Do you "get" him or her? Or is your communication style fraught with misunderstanding?

Listening, talking, and learning to improve our sexual intimacy for the cultivation of oneness in our marriage— that's what the first phase of LEADing to the bedroom is all about. You won't be able to progress to greater intimacy without first understanding where you are and where you want to go. The goal of discovery is not yet to

---

[96] Song of Solomon 1-8.

"fix" anything—simply to understand and be understood. The three primary tasks that increase understanding are:
- Cast vision
- Unearth expectations
- Communicate clearly.

Let's unpack them.

Cast Vision: "I Have a Dream…"

The first law of leading is vision casting—showing people where you want to take them and painting the picture compellingly enough that they want to go with you.

I have great respect for Martin Luther King, Jr.'s leadership, particularly his ability to paint a word picture that powerfully motivates us. As a church planter, I vision cast regularly to our congregation and am always looking to get better at casting a compelling vision.

As a husband and a father, I've also done my share of vision casting. I'm sure you have as well. You are a vision caster if you've ever said anything like:

- "If we save this money, in three years, we'll be able to go on a dream vacation trip."

- "Taking the kids camping will let us spend more time as a family."

- (To your son or daughter) "God will provide the right person for you to marry at the right time. Right now, you let Him make you into the right person."

Each of the statements above has at its core a great dream that, when shared, motivates the hearer to move in that direction. Too often, however, our dreams and vision for our marital intimacy go unshared. When a compelling vision is not cast, your spouse isn't given the opportunity to understand and be motivated to follow the dream. A learning talk with your spouse, is first and foremost, a time of sharing the dream you have for greater intimacy.

Vision casting is really creating a concrete picture of what life would look like if you lived out the values you both share. If you truly value the biblical ideas of "naked and unashamed" oneness[97], joyful sex[98], captivating intimacy[99], sex for protection from temptation[100], etc., it is vital that you each have a concrete picture in your mind of how that looks *today* in your lives, or you'll always trade God's best for the busyness of life.

On the flip side, let me also emphasize what sharing the dream is not. It is *not* placing blame on your spouse for things in the past. In fact, I highly encourage the "sandwich approach" to communicating vision with your spouse. First, praise the things that are in line with your vision for your intimacy. Let her (and him) know what you do like about your intimacy and are thankful for.

Next, for the meat (middle part) of the sandwich, lovingly share what you'd like to be different. Be careful not to put your partner on the defense against you, but do be honest about what should be different for each of you in order to accomplish the dream.

Finally, complete the sandwich with encouragement and praise that you are on the right track and that you are thankful for the progress and foundation you already have. This positioning of the vision (need for change) between authentic encouragement and appreciation ensures that you are not focusing only on the negative. Your spouse needs that.

The vision you cast for your intimacy should be a compelling picture of what you want your relationship to

---

[97] Genesis 2:25.
[98] Song of Solomon 1-8.
[99] Proverbs 5:15-19.
[100] 1 Corinthians 7:1-5.

look like. In order to compel you to move toward it, it must be specific—something you both agree on and can use to guide you as you move forward. At the end of this chapter is a questionnaire to guide your learning talk; it's a useful tool, but don't let it confine your discussion. Take a risk and dream together about what your relationship could be like.

Unearth Expectations: Get on the Same Page

Ah, expectations—we all have them, and in fact, we should. With low expectations, you will both miss God's best plan for your marriage. Particularly as you are learning to LEAD to the bedroom, you should have great expectations that you will have greater intimacy and freedom in your sexual relationship.

But with expectations can come disappointment. When expectations in any area of life are met, there's no problem. You continue on, perhaps even unaware of your expectations. The problem comes when an expectation goes unmet. You had in mind some expectation. Let's say your spouse didn't perform up to some desire you had, be it in courting, sexual frequency, experimentation, etc. The reality didn't meet your expectation, and the gap between what you expected and what you experienced produces feelings of disappointment. The larger the gap, the greater the disappointment.

Figure 12. The Expectation Gap

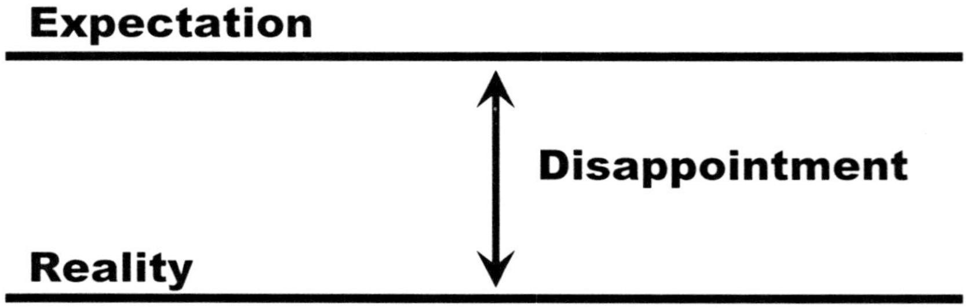

Expectation

Disappointment

Reality

In order to reduce disappointment, then, we can bring reality up to meet expectations, or we can lower our expectations to meet current reality. Which do you think I'd recommend?

The real problem is not the expectation...it's that the enemy has stolen the richness of intimacy God gave us in marriage. I believe most couples can easily raise the current reality they experience and nearly eliminate the disappointment either spouse feels.

In fact, if reality exceeds expectations (in a good way), the resulting feelings are the overwhelming joy and captivation that the lovers in Proverbs 5 and Song of Solomon report. I often ask my bride, "Are you really mine?" It seems too good to be true. When the reality of a loving, giving, need-meeting, oneness-oriented intimate life exceeds your expectations, satisfaction and joy are the result!

I fully believe that almost every Christian marriage is one major adjustment away from captivating joy. What if one vulnerable conversation (or one false belief that is shed, or one action plan, or one commitment to continue toward oneness) is all that's separating you from an overflow of joy instead of a gap of disappointment in your relationship?

Husband, isn't it worth whatever it takes to find out? Wife, won't you follow your husband's lead if it leads to joy? I know you will. But to do it, you've got to unearth the expectations that have been buried—perhaps for years—as the enemy has methodically chipped away at oneness.

Men, when you unearth your expectations and those of your spouse, it is to be loving and supportive. Tell her how beautiful she is, and how much you love her, are pleased by her, and you just want to experience soul oneness with her as God intended for your marriage.

Here's how to get on the same page with your expectations.

Unearthing Expectations

When allowed to stay buried and unexamined, even reasonable and good expectations can cause unexpected stumbling blocks, but God-given expectations that are recognized, owned, encouraged, and vision-casted can help us achieve God's original intent for our marriages.

In order to sort through unmet expectations, there's a helpful process to recognize and clarify your expectations. It's simple but revealing. The first question whenever you (husband or wife) feel frustration should be:

1. *What is my unmet expectation that is causing this emotion?*

You need to identify specifically the expectation you have that is not being met. Consider anger to be an "idiot light," like the warning indicator on your car's dashboard. It's an indicator that an expectation has been unmet. Consciously and concretely state the unmet expectation by completing this sentence:

I expected my spouse to _____.

Once the unmet expectation is identified, the next question is:

2. *Is this a reasonable expectation?*

How do you know if what you're expecting is reasonable? It seems reasonable, or you wouldn't expect it, right? Not so fast. Consider the following ways your expectations might be unreasonable.

Knowledge. Contrary to popular belief, spouses can't read minds. Ladies, sometimes your expectation may be unreasonable because your spouse really doesn't know what you expected unless you tell him. Even if it seems obvious to you, give him the benefit of the doubt—he may need you to spell it out.

Skills, abilities, time, strength, energy, money. Are there hindrances to these or other resources that make yours an unreasonable expectation? When your spouse is tired at the end of the day or when your budget just won't stretch far enough for that romantic getaway, don't expect that your spouse can magically manufacture more resources. We all have limits, and to expect our spouse to go beyond them is unreasonable.

Husbands, sometimes we expect our wives to be superwomen: to work, mother children, keep a neat house, cook dinner, and give their bodies and souls to us— all in the same day. Ask yourself: Is this a reasonable expectation?

God's will. Just to illustrate, if you wanted your spouse to rob a bank to provide for said getaway above, that would be an unreasonable expectation to ask your mate to go against God's will. This could certainly apply to other financial decisions short of a bank heist. Whatever the unmet expectation, ask yourself, does following God's will make this an unreasonable expectation?

If, after considering the possibilities above, you realize your expectation is unreasonable, the right thing to do is to counsel yourself and release the unreasonable expectation from your spouse. It's your problem, not his or hers. Jesus' golden rule is the key here:

Do to others as you would have them do to you.[101]

---

[101] Luke 6:31.

If, on the other hand, your expectation is reasonable, the next question is:

3. Am I demanding that my expectation be met?

It is important to state preferences and dreams, not demands. Demanding goes against the spirit of *agape* love. 1 Corinthians 13 tells us that love is patient and kind…it is not rude, it is not self-seeking, it is not easily angered, it keeps no record of wrongs. The acid test of a demanding spirit is what happens if the expectation is not met: will you exact a price? Anger, pouting, or consequences are all ways of demanding that your expectations be met.

If demanding to get your way is a weakness of yours, ask God to flow his *agape* love through you to your spouse instead.[102]

If you and your spouse are not used to talking about your sex life, it's certain that there are many hopes that are being left unsaid. Both of you likely have unfulfilled expectations in the area of intimacy. Pray and talk with your spouse about your expectations. Work through a solution together. In the "Learning Challenge" at the end of this chapter, you'll find a guide for talking through expectations.

Communicate Clearly: We Need Feedback

I am directionally challenged. You know that sick feeling when you realize you just missed an exit? —I have that feeling all the time. When I drive alone, I allow thirty

---

[102] We learned this model for dealing with expectations from Bob Roland (Fellowship Bible Church, Roswell, GA) in premarital counseling. It has served us well.

extra minutes for the inevitable backtracking I know I'll have to do. If you travel with me, I let you drive.

I used to love Google Maps, the amazing technology that would tell me exactly where to turn, how many miles before my next turn, and step-by-step directions. I thought I was in Heaven. I kept a file of printouts to places I went occasionally.

And it worked well as long as things went perfectly...but throw in a construction detour, a poorly marked intersection, an important mobile phone call— even a brainstorm that comes into my head while I'm driving, and I'm lost again.

Recently though, I discovered the best solution to my navigational woes...GPS! My new best friend in the car tells me out loud that I'm about to miss a turn! But that's not the best part: this little wonder will even recalculate an alternate route for me when I do make a wrong move! That feature must have been created just for me: *"Mr. Reid, you took a wrong turn, but if you'll just go up and make a left, I'll get you back on track without having to turn around."*

Your marriage needs that kind of feedback as well.

Feedback-based Communication

Clear and accurate information is vitally important in navigating unfamiliar roads. Without it, you end up lost and frustrated. Poor communication between spouses about intimacy produces the same result.

There are countless obstacles, pitfalls, and potential sidetracks along the way to your goal of oneness. The stakes are high, so you must give each other feedback to stay on track.

It sounds easy enough, but there's one major problem. We are fallen people in a fallen world under attack by

Satan.[103] And that can make clear communication almost impossible.

We've talked extensively about the enemy and his goals of stealing, killing, and destroying everything good, including soul intimacy. The enemy sends us false ideas about sex and intimacy through movies, culture and advertisements. These work to confuse and shut us down.

But perhaps the hardest part is that our enemy has taken his best shot within our own flesh. Guilt, wounds from the past, insecurity over our bodies, insecurity about leading our wives, fear of following your husbands, and sinful selfishness have made one of God's greatest gifts to humanity also one of the most elusive. We have met the enemy; and they are us.

And if we don't give each other feedback or if we give misleading feedback, we keep going down a wrong turn that leads away from the oneness God intended for us. Let's use some hypothetical navigational pitfalls to illustrate the danger of and the answer to unclear communication in increasing sexual intimacy. Once you recognize these common obstacles to communication and how they may be operating against you, you will likely discover others. You and your spouse probably have your own unique bad habits in communication. Stay alert to remove them before they cause a crash!

Misunderstood Signals

To drive a car, you need to understand the signs on the road. Otherwise, you might end up on a one-way street facing oncoming traffic!

All of us by nature are insecure. (It's directly traceable to the Fall—remember the fig leaves?) And fear and insecurity make us prone to misunderstand any

---

[103] Thank you to Dr. Gary Barnes at Dallas Theological Seminary who gave me this one-sentence summary of the state of the world. It explains so much.

signal from our spouse that is even the slightest bit ambiguous. In especially sensitive situations, important communication often remains unsaid because of fear of rejection. This communication problem in marriage, especially in the area of intimacy, is pandemic.

In fact, a common scenario gets played out over and over in many marriages. Does the following ever (or often) describe your interaction?

A husband asks for intimacy.[104] He receives a less-than-enthusiastic response—a road sign he interprets as "This isn't the time to ask."

Now, in this example scenario, the wife does not mean to send a rejection signal. Likely, she is hesitating for one of two reasons: either she's not feeling good about herself at the moment or she's listening to lies in her mind about what is appropriate sexually.

In fact, it's very likely that what she really wants is to be reassured and pursued, but her signal is misunderstood by her husband in the worst possible way: he thinks she wants to be left alone, and so he does. Many husbands don't even ask anymore because they expect rejection...but they may have just misunderstood the signals.

Wife, if misunderstood signals are your "thing" as a couple (meaning you send each other easily misunderstood signals often), then your husband has been trained by the signals he thinks you've sent him for years to feel that he'll be rejected, so he doesn't ask. Although if he were honest and vulnerable, he'd tell you he wants to be with you far more often than he's comfortable asking. (If you don't believe me, when you're having your learning talk in the right setting, ask him. Husband, don't miss your moment to be understood clearly when she does.)

The effect of misunderstood signals is a complex and inaccurate map we use to navigate our intimate

---

[104] We will consider the "ask" in greater detail in Chapter Six.

relationship. This map is not based on truth, not based on fact, not based on love—but instead based on false perceptions.

Trust me—learning about your mate through prayer and talking is a much better way to establish your expectations and "signals" of your relationship than guesswork. Your spouse won't understand what you really feel without your help.

Read on for two more communication obstacles.

Unwritten Rules

My GPS is generally clear about what it wants to communicate. And road signs can usually be trusted...we know from the time we're three that red means stop and yellow means slow down.

But what if there were rules that your driving teacher forgot to tell you but everyone else on the road seemed to be following? Many couples have unwritten rules that kill the soul sex that God intended. Here are some unintentional and unwritten rules many couples love by and feel bound to even though they don't realize it:

- One or both partners feel they must both climax every time they come together. (Result: inhibits experimentation)
- After a couple comes together, there is an unspoken expectation that they must wait a few days before having sex again. (Result: inhibits frequency, experimentation, and spontaneity)
- One or both partners doesn't feel freedom to satisfy his or her sexual needs to the extent he or she desires, in frequency, variety of position, time of day, etc. (Result: makes sex seem scarce or rigid, which can open the door to frustration and temptation)

If these unwritten rules (or others) are operating in your marriage, they are undoubtedly inhibiting your intimacy. The point is that you didn't agree on these. You might even be hard-pressed to give words to them. But sure enough, they are guidelines for your intimacy, and they aren't helping. What unwritten rules have a strong influence over how you do intimacy, though you've never had a conversation about them? Your learning talk is the time to discuss and evaluate them. Don't let anything hold you back from the oneness God has provided!

Smokescreens

Early in our marriage, when we began to think about buying our first home, I suggested driving around our community to look at houses to get a feel for what we wanted. We hadn't talked price range yet or contacted a real estate agent; this was simply to begin to open our minds to the possibility.

That evening, as we drove by a cute split-level in a ten-year-old neighborhood, I asked Katie what she thought of it. Her answer thoroughly confused me at the time. But our resulting discussion has helped us understand each other better ever since.

She said, "I don't know—a two-story house sounds like too much to clean—can you imagine lugging a vacuum cleaner up and downstairs?" Alarms in my brain went off. No discussion of price, no discussion of square footage, no thought of whether it would be a good investment of our limited money—just "too much to clean."

I immediately begin to make all my counter arguments. And I am good at constructing a case! I told my bride that square footage is a better measure of the size of a house than the number of levels. And if we got a good deal on a two-story house, it would be reasonable to buy an extra vacuum for the upstairs. "One $200 investment is nothing compared to a good deal on a great house that would help us build equity." I remember being particularly proud of this talking point and win for reason and good stewardship.

But the more we talked that night, the further off track my brilliant points got us. Ever had one of those conversations where the more you say, the more distant you feel? Fortunately, though, I began to sense that the vacuum cleaner comment was not really about the economics of two-story houses or about domestic workload. There was something deeper and more important.

> *Ever had one of those talks where the more you say, the more distant you feel?*

So I changed tactics. Instead of debating what *she had said*, I asked gently if perhaps housecleaning wasn't the real issue. She opened up, and thinking through her reaction, she finally concluded, "I'm afraid of the financial responsibility of buying a house—I mean that's something our parents do!"

All my logical reasoning about dual vacuum cleaners was focused on a false target, or a smokescreen. When I realized that my wife was really in need of assurance that we could handle this financially, our conversation took a drastically different (and more productive) turn. We talked about the stability of my job, the soundness of investing in a home appropriate to my income, and the security of trusting God to guide us as we looked for a home.

Often unintentional, a smokescreen is *an alternate idea put forward in the place of the real issue, which the speaker either isn't aware of or is afraid to express.* I believe all couples are prone to smokescreen communication, whether intentional or unintentional, particularly in the sensitive area of intimacy.

What's Behind It?

It is an insightful husband who can look beyond what seems an illogical protest and argument and ask himself, "What does she really mean?" What legitimate fears and concerns may be hiding behind a smokescreen? Perhaps, a wife is not able to put the real issue into words because she doesn't even know what the real issue is. What better way to grow closer than to sensitively help identify what is holding both of you back from greater oneness?

Getting past the smokescreens in your conversation is one of the most productive things you can do for your marriage. When an objection does not make sense to me, I tell Katie, "This sounds like a smokescreen. (We use this term lovingly, so it is not offensive.) Can we help each other figure out what the real issue is?" Getting on the same team sure beats arguing the wrong case.

Solomon and his bride's intimate relationship is a great example of a lack of smokescreens. He speaks candidly to her; she's frank and forward with him about what she desires and needs.[105] You can be that bold and vulnerable with each other when you have a protective wall of unconditional love around your relationship.

Do you think there are some smokescreens in your marriage in the area of intimacy? I'd bet there are. One of you needs to stop creating a smokescreen; the other needs to keep pursuing.

The Learning Challenge

We've introduced several communication concepts in this chapter, everything from casting vision, unearthing buried expectations, and communicating clearly with your mate. Now, it's time to apply these concepts to your

---

[105] Song of Solomon 4:15-16, 6:4-7, 7:1-8:4, and 8:13-14, among others. They unashamedly describe each other's attractiveness and their desire for sex.

relationship with your first learning talk. Here's how to do it.

In one to two hours (quit while you are ahead), use the questions below to guide your learning talk. Don't try to answer them all; focus only on the areas that seem important to you. It can get overwhelming if you try to cover too much. The goal is to have multiple learning talks over time, perhaps a monthly talk to review recent progress and tackle new issues in bite-sized chunks.

This conversation may very well delve into uncharted territory for you. Push through the initial awkwardness that will accompany this new vulnerable expression, and resist the urge not to "go there." If approached in a spirit of faith, hope, and love, the fruit of your learning talk will be deeper understanding, and the more talks you have, the better they will be. Give your spouse permission to be completely honest.

At the end of your first learning talk, you should be able to briefly state a shared vision, articulate expectations that are currently unmet, and identify poor communication tendencies in your relationship with some ideas of how to correct them. Don't feel overwhelmed if there are many barriers to oneness right now. The point of the learning talk is to get it all out on the table—to discover where you are. There are still three steps to go to LEAD to the bedroom.

Suggested Learning Talk Questions

Cast Vision: I Have a Dream...
1. Where do you want to go with your intimacy? (What do you value?)
2. What do you dream of in the area of courtship and sex?
   a. Describe your perfect romantic night (paint the picture, including many details like having a romantic dinner (in or out), your spouse meeting you at the door, giving you full attention, etc.)
   b. How often would you like to be together sexually?
   c. What kind of variety would you like to add to your sex life?
   d. What would make you feel more passion?
3. What would be a dream date for you? (Give a couple of examples.)

Unearth Expectations: Let's Get on the Same Page
1. What do you like that we are currently doing?
2. What do you not like?
3. What do you want in the future?
4. Would you be willing to _____? (Fill in the blank with something you want to do, but have been too shy to ask.)
5. What expectations do you have that I am not meeting?
6. Do you make your expectations in the following areas known?
   a. Courting
   b. Frequency
   c. Fun
   d. Erotic Fantasies

Feedback-Based Communication
Misunderstood Signals
1. Each partner should ask the other these questions (and consider whether your signals are being properly understood).
   "What signals do you think I send to you about..."
   - a. Agape Commitment
   - b. Frequency
   - c. Fun/Freedom
   - d. Passion/Romance
   - e. When it's okay to initiate intimacy
2. When I ask for intimacy, how do you respond? Am I sorry I asked? (Is this misunderstood?)
3. What is often misunderstood in our communication about our intimacy?
4. Do you think it is a sending or receiving problem (or both)?
5. How could we change that?

Unwritten Rules
1. What are your unwritten rules? (e.g., We must both climax every time we come together, or we must wait a few days before having sex again.)
2. Is there a great intimate experience you can remember that you've never felt open enough to ask for again? Is there an "unwritten rule" that keeps you from asking?
3. What if one of your new rules (spoken aloud and agreed to) was, "It's alright (in fact, it's awesome!) to try new things." How would that make you feel (husband, then wife)? Why not decide that together?

Smokescreens
1. What smokescreens are hindering us from greater oneness?
2. Can we put them into words today and get on the same team?

Chapter Five
E – Experience the Gospel
Repent & Believe

"The time has come," Jesus said. "The kingdom of God is near. Repent and believe the good news!"

—Mark 1:15

Sex is only 10% of a good marriage, but it's 90% if it's not going right.

—Author Unknown

"I'm sorry...I am not a sexpot!" Katie's response effectively shut down the conversation and my attempt to express my desire for more adventurous intimacy. As God began to show me months later how to LEAD in the area of intimacy, I wrote this to her about her statement.

Looking back, that day was very sorrowful for me. Out of insecurity, you were repeating one of Satan's lies: "I can't give you what you need." I also heard, "I won't try, and you shouldn't ask me."

I realize that in my private thoughts I grieve the absence of the kind of soul sexual intimacy that God created a wife to have with her husband. In my efforts to be a loving husband—as well as dealing with my own insecurities about feeling rejected if I ask—I now recognize you have no idea about many of the deep desires I have on an ongoing basis.

I live life secretly hoping perhaps today you'll want to be in the shower together, linger in the tub, or try a score of sensual ideas I'd love to share with you. I believe we are meant to <u>both</u> enjoy a whole other level of uninhibited sexual intimacy together.

I pray you will realize that you can provide all the soul-touching intimacy I crave. Everything about you: your gorgeous body, your feminine ways, your stimulating mind, your heart for God, your personality, and your partnership with me in all of life—they all cry out for me to take you however I desire with wild abandon like Solomon and his bride. She welcomed it as I wish you could. The one thing against us is the lie that you can't provide soul-stirring intimacy to your husband.

A Wife's Take

I'll never forget that day...I really so wanted David to pursue me, and yet I had just pushed him away big time. We were really mixed up then. I said the opposite of what I really wanted so many times before we committed to work together to pursue greater intimacy in our relationship.

Nowhere does God's Word use the term "sexpot" to describe the sexuality of a wife. (I have no idea where I picked that up!) But it does say wonderful things like:

- "your love is better than wine," (Song 4:10)
- "may her breasts satisfy you always," (Proverbs 5:19a)
- "may you ever be captivated by her love," (Proverbs 5:19b), and
- the wife is the "fountain" of sexuality for her husband (Proverbs 5:15-18).

These truths about how we were created are so often lost in the din of lies from the world, the Devil, and our own fleshly insecurities. My prayer as you read this chapter is that you will truly experience God's good news for your intimate life.

A million things can go wrong in a marriage, and intimacy is often a major casualty. However, we have a God who specializes in redeeming lost and damaged people—and marriages.

> *We have a God who specializes in redeeming damaged marriages.*

Experiencing the Gospel is the most powerful step in LEADing to the bedroom. Paul said that the gospel is the "power of God for salvation to everyone who believes."[106] In his context, the gospel is the good news that Jesus has come to earth to set right everything that has gone wrong with the world as a result of the Fall.

In American evangelicalism, we tend to think of the "gospel" in the very narrow sense of Jesus' death, burial, and resurrection on the third day[107] that "whoever believes in Him will not perish, but have eternal life."[108]

Certainly, God's good news (the meaning of the word "gospel") has as its source and greatest expression the truth that we are no longer destined to Hell if we put our trust in Christ because Jesus defeated death through His crucifixion and Resurrection. However, in Romans, Paul defines the gospel with much greater present-life implication than is often preached. The "full life" Jesus promised in John 10:10 starts now and encompasses the redeeming power of Christ in every sphere of our life.

So, while being true to the Scriptures, let me expand our definition of the gospel and reveal the glorious implications it has for marriage. The gospel, in a broader sense, is really all of God's good news for His creation. This includes the truth that God put one man and one woman together in marriage for greater joy and oneness.

---

[106] Romans 1:16.
[107] 1 Corinthians 15:1-4.
[108] John 3:16.

The Gospel with Respect to Sex

Specifically, the aspect of God's good news I want to emphasize is the Creation passage:

"And the man and his wife were both naked and were not ashamed."[109]

God intended husbands and wives to be completely vulnerable with each other (sexually) and have no shame. That's good news for us! That's part of God's gospel.

But, the most powerful part of the good news is this: though God's enemy tried to wreck everything good about His creation (beginning in Genesis 3 and continuing today), Jesus came with power to redeem and deliver us from the enemy's sabotage. In John 10:10b, Jesus says He came that we "might have life, and life to the full." This isn't just eternal life, but a full and abundant life starting now. This absolutely covers the restoration of God-blessed sex as a catalyst to greater oneness as it was meant to be in the Garden.[110]

A Two-Part Process

The New Testament is clear about how to experience God's good news in our life by receiving salvation and growing in holiness, including experiencing God's best and wholeness in the area of married sex.

The Scriptures often speak of experiencing the gospel as a two-part process. Consider these verses:

"The time has come," he said. *"The kingdom of God is near. **Repent** and **believe** the good news!"*
                                                   —Mark 1:15

---

[109] Genesis 2:25.
[110] Ultimately, Jesus will bring about a complete return to the beauty and peace of the Garden in Genesis 2. All in due time.

When Jesus announced His ministry in Mark 1, He called for two things: repentance and belief.

The kingdom of God is near. Repent and believe the Good News.

I have declared to both Jews and Greeks that they must turn to God in **repentance** *and* **have faith** *in our Lord Jesus.*

—Acts 20:21

Here, in Paul's farewell to the elders of Ephesus, he summarizes his ministry among them as speaking the dual message of repentance and faith in Jesus.

Finally, look at the recurring theme of repentance and belief in Paul's letters:

You were taught, with regard to your former way of life, to **put off your old self,** *[repent] which is being corrupted by its deceitful desires;* **to be made new in the attitude of your minds;** *and to* **put on the new self,** *[believe] created to be like God in true righteousness and holiness.*

—Ephesians 4:22-24[111]

Paul tells us to put off our sinful nature and put on the new one by changing our beliefs. Again, there is this two-step process. Off with the old, on with the new.

In a foundational passage you may have memorized, Paul encapsulated these two steps in one verse:

Do not conform *any longer to the pattern of this world, but* **be transformed by the renewing of your mind.** *Then you will be able to test and*

---

[111] See also Romans 13:12-14 and Colossians 3:8-10 where Paul uses "put off" and "put on" terminology to describe repentance and belief.

approve what God's will is—his good, pleasing and perfect will.

—Romans 12:2

What he is saying is repent (change the old way you think that is false) and believe God's good news.

...be transformed by the renewing of your mind.

Getting Rid of Your Junk

Katie loves interior decorating TV shows. I tolerate them. However, one does intrigue me. Aptly called *Clean House,* it's a "design on a dime" show with one really interesting twist...the people chosen for the show are all pack rats. I mean, can't-walk-for-all-the-junk-in-my-house pack rats. And here's the kicker: in order to have money for the remodel, you have to sell your old junk. Did you get that? **You've got to get rid of your old junk before you can have the new life you want.**

Oh, they fight it! The design team, especially the colorful hostess, pleads, begs, and threatens the homeowners to let go of their clutter and tasteless furnishings.

This illustrates what repentance is all about. On the show, the more they repent (change their thinking) and let go of their falsely held beliefs (that their stuff is worth keeping), the more improvement they end up with.

You've got to get rid of your old junk before you have room for the new life you want.

The Greek word *metanoeo* (repent) is often confused with changing your outward behaviors alone (works). Biblically, it actually means to change your *mind*, that is, to change the way you *think* about something, which then affects your whole person, as new thinking informs new ways of living which become habits.

Repentance (this change of thinking) is the first step in salvation or in sanctification (or in the specialized area of experiencing God's good news in our sex life).

In salvation, it means to turn away from the faulty thinking you had:
- you are not sinful,
- what you think is right,
- you should control your life

so that you can believe the truth:
- you are sinful,
- you need a Savior, and
- Jesus is the omnipotent God of the universe Who loves you enough that He sacrificed Himself to meet your need. The only thing that makes sense is to surrender your life to Him. He should lead your life.

Repent and believe is like the old computer-programming rule, GIGO. If you put Garbage In, you'll get Garbage Out. So the first step to a true spiritual relationship with God is to change our thinking from our false beliefs to God's truth.

As we grow in Christ, all of our maturing continues this process of repenting (changing our thinking) and believing God's good news (learning that we can fully trust Him). We learn to repent and believe in the areas of money, pride, parenting, relationships—everything. As we change our false thinking and begin to believe and trust in Jesus, we are more usable by God, and we experience the full life Jesus promised in John 10:10. We are meant to experience this same sanctifying process in our sexual intimacy.

We are meant to experience this same sanctifying process in our sexual intimacy.

Repent (Change the Way You Think About Sex)

Experiencing the gospel in your sex life begins with changing your false thoughts and beliefs about sex. Don't underestimate the importance of "cleaning house" of your false beliefs, the lies the enemy has told you. In the words of the *Clean House* hostess: *Honey, we're gonna' get rid of some of your junk today!*

> *Experiencing the gospel in your sex life begins with changing your false beliefs about sex.*

Here's how: first, ask Jesus to reveal to you what lies you need to stop believing, and ask God and your spouse to help you in this process. You will most likely need his or her help to identify the lies you believe.

In order to deal with the false, sinful, or hindering beliefs and thought patterns that shape your intimacy, let's address husbands and wives separately. But first, we need to establish an important guideline for this sensitive realm.

Collaboration

Convincing your partner to repent is not your job, it's the Holy Spirit's—and you want to give Him ample room to work. Experiencing the gospel is a work of God in the life of each partner, or it's nothing.

> *Convincing your partner to repent is not your job, it's the Holy Spirit's.*

An all-important key to experiencing the gospel is that each of you willingly examines yourself and your "stuff." Let God deal with your spouse. Spirit-led conviction can do what years of nagging or complaining only hinder. If you are serious about focusing on your issues and doing your part, He will make it clear when and how you can help your partner.

So, what is your role in this process? Your learning talk should have yielded some honest and insightful truths about the state of your intimacy. Start there in your own heart. Individually work through the following

Repent and *Believe* sections first. Then it will be time to collaborate, which is the very heart of oneness.

Repentance for Husbands

Husband, what do you need to repent of? Read these carefully and prayerfully and check all that apply to you.[112]

Potential False Beliefs or Actions for a Husband to Repent of

Body Image

_____I am insecure about my body and sexuality.

_____I have not valued myself, therefore I haven't taken care of my body.

Deficient View of Sex

_____I thought a sexy wife would be one who felt and responded sexually just like I did as a man.

_____I angrily believed the lie that my wife never wanted sex when she simply said, "Not tonight."

_____I need to repent of settling for the lowest common denominator[113] in our intimacy.

_____I have allowed pornography or lust to steal oneness with my wife.

_____I have allowed pornography and worldly culture to define exciting sex and robbed my wife of her own unique sexiness.

_____I have obsessed over some sexual behavior and let it get in the way of true, intimate lovemaking.

------

[112] I encourage you to treat this as a checklist to prioritize what false thinking you specifically need to repent of. You can download a free Repent and Believe worksheet at www.leadingtothebedroom.com.

[113] The lowest common denominator is the minimum amount of intimacy both partners agree on, as opposed to aiming for the greatest level of intimacy possible (see Chapter Three).

Deficient View of Oneness

_____I have not been leading in the area of intimacy, so I'm allowing us to miss the blessing we could have.

_____I do not share my whole heart and desires with my wife.

_____I do not court my wife in a way that communicates love and absolute acceptance and appreciation for her (touches her soul).

_____I have allowed the enemy to steal the depth of soul oneness the Lord intended to give us.

_____I go passive instead of leading in the area of intimacy.

_____I get angry instead of lovingly leading my wife to greater oneness.

_____I think of oneness in terms of sex only, not in terms of relating to my wife emotionally.

_____I have falsely assumed my wife had low sexual desire when she was actually tired and emotionally disconnected.

_____I think of oneness as sex or emotional closeness, but not in terms of helping with the kids or around the house.

_____I think of marriage as 50/50 (you owe me your part) instead of unconditional commitment regardless of what my wife does.

_____I've been rejected so many times, I'm afraid of rejection.

_____I need to repent of abdicating leadership.

_____I need to repent of selfishly wanting my own needs met regardless of my wife's feelings.

_____In frustration, I have shut down emotionally.

_____I've neglected to cherish my wife, providing her with fulfillment through romance and affection.

_____I forget that my wife's emotional needs are different. She needs me to give my heart and soul to her through conversation.

_____I sometimes take advantage of my role as leader by being bossy and demanding.

_____I am sexually and emotionally self-focused at times and not a servant.

_____I focus on my "rights" instead of my responsibilities.

_____I fail to ask about and listen to my wife's desire and need for greater intimacy.

_____I sometimes ignore or am lazy about my wife's desire and need for romantic gestures.

_____I have allowed work responsibilities/fatigue to be an excuse for neglecting my responsibilities as a husband and a father.

Deficient View of God

_____I do not trust that Jesus has the power to guide our relationship back to the fullness of Genesis 2.

_____Other:_____

_____

Repentance for Wives

Ladies, what do you need to repent of? Often, much of the repentance a wife needs to do is to turn away from lies the enemy has told her. Read these carefully and prayerfully, and check all that apply to you.

Potential False Beliefs or Actions for a Wife to Repent of

Body Image

_____I don't think I'm beautiful/desirable/sexy.

_____I have deep insecurity about my body and sexuality.

_____I have not valued myself, therefore I haven't taken care of my body.

Deficient View of Sex

_____I feel awkward talking about our intimacy, so I shut my husband down when he brings it up.

_____I have an idea that sex with my husband is somehow dirty, especially if it involves more adventurous aspects.

_____I don't expect to be able to enjoy sex as much as my husband.

_____I struggle at a deep, almost subconscious level thinking that sex with my husband is a "duty," rather than recognizing it as a God-ordained joy, comfort, and catalyst to greater oneness.

_____I have not been assertive in telling my husband what I enjoy or desire sexually in our lovemaking.

_____I have allowed the media to dictate my view of sex.

_____I have emotional baggage that is holding me back.

Deficient View of Oneness

_____I don't realize that I am the only one who can provide my husband with physical and mental sexual fulfillment/release/satisfaction in a godly way.

_____I sometimes forget that part of my God-given role is to keep my husband from being tempted to meet his needs for physical and emotional closeness in another way.[114]

_____I often respond negatively when my husband asks for sex.

_____I have not developed helpful ways of postponing sex and being able to graciously suggest another time.

_____I fear that if I share my body willfully, my husband will become demanding and want more than I can give.

_____I am sometimes shy with my husband.

_____I don't intentionally think about sex enough and reserve energy for lovemaking.

_____I discourage my husband from leading by my attitude or actions.

_____I need to decide to encourage and engage my husband in intimate conversations when he leads us to sexual topics.

_____I need to recognize that sex isn't merely a physical need for my husband but an emotional one, also—that it is directly related to his feelings of manhood, adequacy, and self-esteem.

---

[114] 1 Corinthians 7:1-5.

_____I base my sexual response to my husband on my feelings of the moment rather than a commitment and choice to give.

_____I withhold sex to manipulate or punish.

Deficient View of God

_____I don't trust that Jesus has the power to guide our relationship back to the fullness of Genesis 2.

_____I don't think I can provide soul-stirring sexual intimacy to my husband. (Ultimately, this is thinking that reflects a deficient view of God.)

_____Other:_____

_____

It's very possible that the above lists are discouraging, perhaps even overwhelming, as you realize the lies of the enemy you have believed, the real scars you bear from life in a fallen world, and the weaknesses of your own flesh that have robbed you of the intimacy God intended to bless your marriage. It's sobering to realize that you aren't where you dreamed you'd be—and downright painful if you have lost hope of getting there.

But don't forget the point of this chapter. There is *good news* when Jesus comes into the picture. He came to give life, and life to the fullest.

So, now go back through your list and consciously repent of your false thinking. Read the statements that you checked, and reject each of them as a lie or sin. Make a conscious decision that you are "taking out the trash" to use our *Clean House* analogy.

Biblically speaking, you are repenting: doing an about-face in your *thinking*—turning away from the lies you believe so that you can embrace God's good news for you.

It's probable that the enemy has whispered these lies to you for a lifetime—and your flesh is, after all, fleshly—so you must be intentional about changing your thinking. Take your top three or top one false beliefs/actions above and make it a daily matter to talk to God and your spouse about. That leads us to the husband's unique role.

The Husband's Role in Experiencing the Gospel

You cannot lead where you will not go. Husband, you need to lead in repentance—before you can lead your wife to change her false thinking, you must change yours. I know it seems like a bold, possibly even arrogant, stance to help your wife identify in what areas she needs to repent (change her thinking), especially when you know how you fail.

Start with yourself. Honestly analyze your thinking, and then "speaking the truth in love", you'll be able to humbly help your wife begin to address her list with prayer and conversation.

This is vital because our enemy's time-tested sabotage is getting the husband to abdicate leadership. It's there when God's Word says, "she also gave [the fruit] to her husband, who was with her, and he ate it."[115] It's there when a husband says today, "I'm not perfect, so what right do I have to talk?"

> *Our Enemy's time-tested sabotage is getting the husband to abdicate leadership.*

Don't give in to the enemy's trick! Lead by example. Boldly and humbly confess the lies you listen to and the sin you commit. Then humbly help your wife do the same. God designed her to respond to leadership like that; you'll see—if you're willing to try it.

This kind of leading is not a demand but an invitation. When done as Christ loves the church, you are

---

[115] Genesis 3:6.

saying to your wife, "I will be gentle, patient, understanding, longsuffering, and forgiving, but I can no longer abdicate leadership in an area so vital to the joy and oneness we can have and were meant to experience." You are like Solomon leading his bride toward greater oneness (and joyful sex) with the invitation to "Arise my beloved, and come away with me."[116]

The Second Step: Believe

In the 1850s, Charles Blondin repeatedly traversed 1100 feet of tightrope 170 feet above the ground across Niagara Falls. He was a showman, sometimes pushing a wheelbarrow across the chasm to emphasize his great balance. After completing the death-defying walk, he would call out, "Do you believe I can do this again?" to electrify the spectators.

The crowd would go wild: "Yes, we believe you can do it, Charles!"

"Then, get in!" Charles motioned toward the empty wheelbarrow. Suddenly the crowd would become quiet.

What does it mean to believe? Just as with repentance, the word *believe* (or *pisteuo* in the Greek) is often misunderstood. While we think of it as mental assent or agreement with a set of facts, it actually means to commit your trust to something or someone, as in the case of believing in Jesus (or getting in the wheelbarrow).

So, biblically, believing the gospel goes beyond mere agreement with this statement:

I believe Jesus was a real person who died on the Cross and was raised the third day.

We must actually depend on (trust) the truth God has for us:

---

[116] Song of Solomon 2:10.

I trust Jesus as God. Jesus, You control the entire universe. You're all-powerful, all-knowing, and all-wise. And You...love...me. You proved it by dying on the cross to pay for my sin. I now rely on you (and nothing else) as the only way to Heaven and a full life here and now. Your Resurrection proves You have the power to overcome any obstacle, and therefore, I will fully rely on You instead of my thinking and my striving. I surrender my life over to You to lead. Jesus, You are my Savior (who died and rose again to give me forgiveness of sin) and my Lord (the master/leader of my life).

That's the gospel! And that's why I much prefer the word *trust* to express the biblical idea of faith **Biblical belief is a trust that leads to surrender.** and belief—you're actually trusting your life to Jesus and not just agreeing with a set of facts about Him. Belief in Jesus that saves you goes beyond mere assent into surrender and dependence on Him. If you really get who Jesus is and what He did for you, nothing else but an initial surrender of your life to Him, followed by a lifetime of learning to trust Him more, even makes sense.

If you haven't yet trusted Christ as the italicized paragraph above indicates, I invite you to make it your prayer right now. Trusting Christ with your life is the most important decision you will ever make.[117]

Having cleaned out your false thinking, you need to get in the wheelbarrow and trust Jesus to carry you across the gap to greater intimacy. Do you believe that He can do it? Personally, I find it much easier to trust Christ than to think about getting in Blondin's wheelbarrow.

---

[117] If you just trusted Christ, congratulations! I would love to celebrate with you and help you get started in your new life with Jesus. My contact info can be found at the end of this book.

Read on to find out the good news He has for you.

Believe the Gospel (God's Good News)

God has *lots* of good news about sex in marriage. Following is a primer of good news to believe: first general truth, then spouse-specific. I can't stress how important it is for your future progress in intimacy to repent of old thinking patterns and false beliefs and to trust and fully believe the good news God has for you in the area of intimacy.

Carefully consider each of the following truth statements derived from God's Word regarding marital intimacy. Check any that are particularly difficult for you to believe (rely on as true in your life).

Good News to Believe

Good News about Jesus

I have come that they may have life, and have it to the full. —John 10:10

_____1. Believe Jesus came to give us abundant life, including soul sex that is deeply satisfying to both partners and a catalyst for greater oneness.

Everything is possible for him who believes. —Mark 9:23

_____2. Believe that Jesus is able to increase your intimacy as the husband leads his wife and she grows in giving her husband more of herself and her husband in giving more of himself.

I can do everything through Him who gives me strength. —Philippians 4:13

_____3. Believe Jesus *can* heal each spouse's wound that Satan has used to steal intimacy from your marriage.

_____4. Believe the Lord can make a way for *whatever* you need (more romantic dating, for instance).

Good News about Sex

The man and his wife were both naked, and they felt no shame. —Genesis 2:25

_____5. Sexual intimacy in marriage is good.

_____6. Sexual intimacy is designed by God.

_____7. Sex is meant to be a blessing.

_____8. Sex is needed by husband and wife to warm up the whole relationship.

_____9. Sexual intimacy is not shameful to talk about. (Even if you didn't have a great first learning talk, you need to believe this.)

...put [your] hope in God, who richly provides us with everything for our enjoyment. —1 Timothy 6:17

_____10. Sex is a gift from God for enjoyment.

_____11. Sex is designed to be a catalyst for greater oneness.

...may her breasts satisfy you always,
may you ever be captivated by her love.
Why be captivated, my son, by an adulteress?
Why embrace the bosom of another man's wife? —Proverbs 5:19-20

_____12. In order to meet the purposes in #10 and #11, sex is meant to be varied, passionate, frequent, fun, abandoned, uninhibited, sensual, and erotic. (Genesis, Song of Solomon, Proverbs, and 1 Corinthians 7 affirm that sex in marriage is good.)

_____13. Scripture affirms that anything in the marriage bed that promotes oneness between a married couple is permissible and good (Proverbs 5, Song of Solomon, Hebrews 13:4).

The husband should fulfill his marital duty to his wife, and likewise the wife to her husband. The wife's body does not belong to her alone but also to her husband. In the same way, the husband's body does not belong to him alone but also to his wife.   —1 Corinthians 7:3-4

_____14. The husband and wife do not own their bodies any more, but have given themselves to their partner. If one partner wants something that he or she feels would promote oneness, the other has a covenant obligation to consider their partner's requests. (It may sound like I'm talking only about sex, but this also applies to conversation, conflict resolution, date nights, etc.)

_____15. There is NOTHING dirty or shameful about a husband and wife enjoying each other's bodies passionately and fully. This includes such things as variety of position, oral sex, fully abandoning your body to your husband (or wife), giving up control and relaxing so you can enjoy your spouse pleasuring you.

_____16. Also, part of the good news is that marriage (as well as other aspects of the Christian life) requires discipline born of submission to the Holy Spirit in order to mature. In order to achieve greater oneness, we must treat our sex lives as a blessing to be nurtured and grown, just as important as growing in the area of good stewardship. (Saying that oneness and selflessness take work may not seem like good news, but the great news is that God provides a Helper, the Holy Spirit, who makes selfless marriage and true oneness possible.)

_____17. Couples are meant to *share* their deepest thoughts, feelings, and romantic/erotic fantasies in order to promote exclusive oneness. That is the unique blessing of marriage. (Note Solomon's conversations with his bride.)

_____18. A great sex life is a gift of God to pursue.

_____19. Married sex is a protection against temptation to lust.[118]

God's Good News for Husbands

_____20. You as the husband are ordained by God to be the leader (head) in marriage (Eph. 5:23). This includes leading in the area of intimacy. You are called to be bold and confident, to lead to greater levels of intimacy and oneness and not let Satan steal what God ordained for couples to have.

_____21. Believe that Jesus has the power to help you become a gentle servant leader with the ability to get beyond your own selfishness and wisely influence change.

_____22. Believe that God can help you understand, relate well with, and fully express your heart to your wife.

_____23. Believe that God can and wants to redeem your marriage, no matter what ups and downs you've been through.

God's Good News for Wives

_____24. You are not a "sexpot" – you are your husband's "fountain," a spring of overflowing beauty and passion and sexual refreshment to fully satisfy your husband's thirst for **you**.[119]

---

[118] 1 Corinthians 7:5.
[119] Proverbs 5:15-20.

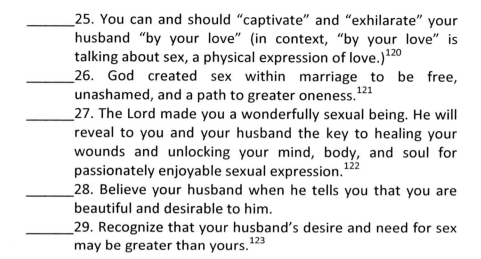

_____25. You can and should "captivate" and "exhilarate" your husband "by your love" (in context, "by your love" is talking about sex, a physical expression of love.)[120]

_____26. God created sex within marriage to be free, unashamed, and a path to greater oneness.[121]

_____27. The Lord made you a wonderfully sexual being. He will reveal to you and your husband the key to healing your wounds and unlocking your mind, body, and soul for passionately enjoyable sexual expression.[122]

_____28. Believe your husband when he tells you that you are beautiful and desirable to him.

_____29. Recognize that your husband's desire and need for sex may be greater than yours.[123]

Which truths above are hard for you to believe? There may be some you either don't understand or aren't sure about. You must be convinced of their truth, or you will never be able to believe them. For the ones you have questions about, seek out the answers you are looking for. Reread Chapter Two: Soul Sex, talk to a trusted pastor, study your Bible, read a commentary on the Scripture passages we've cited often, check out the additional resources in the back of this book, and, certainly, ask the Holy Spirit to "guide you into all truth."[124]

But don't dismiss a statement out of hand because it doesn't "sit well" with you or because it hasn't seemed true in the past. That's exactly how the enemy wants to keep hidden from you the "full life" Jesus came to give you.

For other statements that you are struggling with (but don't question if they are true), take the top three or

---

[120] Proverbs 5:19. It is interesting that "captivate" is the same word as "intoxicate."

[121] Genesis 2:25.

[122] Luke 11:9-10.

[123] 1 Corinthians 7:1-5.

[124] John 16:13.

top one (if it's a big one), and write them in your journal as a daily matter of prayer. Write out the truth with a Scripture reference and put it on your bathroom mirror to meditate on.[125]

Jesus did come to give you a full life, including great intimacy in your marriage. Christ in you can accomplish the needed

> **For the Bathroom Mirror:**
> **My husband thinks I'm**
> **hot. – Proverbs 5:15-19**

changes in your marriage. Your job is to clean out your false thinking and believe the good news of Jesus. That's change from the inside out, and it is the only lasting change. You have a lifetime of lies in your head; give God some time to affirm the truth and write it on your heart.

Now that you've worked through these truth statements alone, set a time soon to have an honest conversation with your spouse.[126] Read on for how to do this.

Prepare to Die!

Before you have your next learning talk, you need to prepare to die—to your old way of thinking. At its core, the gospel actually requires that we die to the sinful nature we were born with so that Christ may live His pure and sinless life through us.

The wonderful byproduct is that He gives us inexplicable joy despite our circumstances, and all we trade for it in return is the punishment we deserved for sinning against a Holy God. This is God's grace (unearned favor), and it is the deal of a lifetime for us![127]

---

[125] Philippians 4:8.

[126] Refer back to the previous chapter for a reminder of how to create a good setting for an intimate conversation.

[127] If you have not trusted Jesus as your Savior, you need to acknowledge that you are a sinner in need of God's grace, believe that Jesus died on the Cross to take away your sin, and begin to trust that He can lead your life better than you can. Pray to tell Him that is your heart's desire. (You might want to use the

Paul puts it like this in another place:

Therefore, if anyone is in Christ, he is a new creation; the old has gone, the new has come![128]

It is perfectly clear that new life comes from dying to something old. God wants you to die to your old way of doing intimacy, your old way of having sex, your old way of quid pro quo instead of generosity leading to total oneness with your spouse. Sound impossible? The truth is that with Jesus' power, He'll do through us what we can't do for ourselves.

Experience the Gospel Together

Husband, you should lovingly lead through this next conversation. Begin by praying for God to work in you and move you both toward greater oneness. Ask God to stop the enemy from his attempts to destroy your current effort to grow closer together.

Next, tell your wife what the Holy Spirit has shown you that you need to repent of (either from the repentance list or other self-examination) and which new truths need to replace your false thinking.

My brother, this is your moment. Don't do like our Grandpa Adam and stay silent when you should speak up. Don't abdicate your God-ordained leadership. You have the benefit of knowing where that leads, and you have the Holy Spirit to help you.

Your wife is wired to respond to honesty and servant leadership. Don't just read the sentence off the page. Look into her eyes and tell her why you realize you need to

italicized prayer on p. 132 as a guide.) If you just trusted Christ, I'd love to celebrate with you and help you get started in your new life with Jesus. My contact info can be found at the end of this book.

[128] 2 Corinthians 5:17.

repent of or believe a certain statement. Give illustrations. Tell her the insight you felt as the light came on in a specific area. Intimacy is not only in the bedroom. It's right now as you talk. Eloquence does not matter. You may have never been this vulnerable with your wife in your life, but this could be the very key to your wife's heart.

Wife, be supportive. The subject matter is already sensitive, and now your husband is talking with you about areas in which he's failed and needs to change. This is holy ground. How you respond has a huge impact on how he'll share with you now and in the future. Don't interject until he's finished.

But husband, the ball is really in your court. You are called by God to be the leader. Love her as Christ loved the church. If you blow it, apologize, regroup your thoughts, and try again. If she makes a mistake and the conversation goes badly, you need to forgive first, love unconditionally, and work to pick up the pieces and restore the relationship. (Think about Jesus going to the Cross while we were still sinners.[129]) You know that our enemy is really Satan, who is trying at every turn to steal, kill, and destroy. So help you God, that will not happen in your marriage. Men, don't stop leading in a godly way.

Next, wives should share what the Lord has shown them they need to repent of and believe. Men, don't blow this. This is perhaps the most vulnerable your wife has ever been with you. Future oneness depends on you not being an oaf. (I speak from experience.)

Men, future oneness depends on you not being an oaf.

Each of you should "speak the truth in love"[130] and encourage each other regarding progress. Use the

---

[129] Romans 5:8.
[130] Ephesians 4:15.

sandwich[131] method of praise/correction/praise when either of you wants to encourage your partner to change his or her thinking even more.

Work at listening without the need to defend or "fix." No matter how insignificant or purely emotional something may sound to you at first, don't judge. This is not you vs. me, but us (with Jesus) vs. the world, the flesh, and the Devil. Hear your mate's heart so you can join together in the real fight.

Discern how long the conversation should last, men. It is better to quit while you are ahead and wanting to talk more than to wish you had stopped earlier. I recommend you keep this round of "Repent and Believe" conversation to under an hour. These discussions will get easier and more fruitful the more often you have them. So, part of your goal is to end on a positive note.

As you finish, commit to encouraging and reminding each other (gently) to reject false thinking and replace it with the good news of Christ. Husbands, close the meeting by praying tenderly for your wives. Thank God for His good news for your marriage. Ask Him to help you both repent and believe the gospel with respect to your intimacy.

Ladies, it would encourage your husband greatly if you prayed aloud also, thanking God for a courageous husband who leads and telling God in front of your husband that you are committed to following his lead and blessing him as you grow in believing the gospel.

Review

We've covered a lot of material in this chapter about the most powerful part of LEADing to the Bedroom. So that we don't risk missing the forest for the trees, let me

---

[131] This sandwich method is described in the previous chapter.

summarize this step, *Experience the Gospel*, before we proceed to put it into action in the next chapter.

The gospel is God's good news in all its fullness. It includes the transforming power of Jesus Christ to work in our lives—even in our sexual intimacy, which the enemy has been working to systematically destroy ever since the Fall in Genesis 3.

The key to experiencing God's good news in our lives is two-fold: repent (of false thinking) and believe (trust) in God's truth. Romans 12:2 says to "be transformed by the *renewing of your mind*." Ephesians 4:22-24 instructs us to "put off" our [old nature] and "put on" our [new nature]. In the context of our intimacy, it looks like this:

Repent	Believe
Husbands, put off	**Husbands, put on**
Dependence on our flesh	Dependence on Christ
Passivity	Leadership
Insecurity	Confidence in Christ
Domination	Servant Attitude
And so on...	And so on...
Wives, put off	**Wives, put on**
Dependence on our flesh	Dependence on Christ
Insecurity	Confidence in Christ
Feelings of inferiority	Belief in your God-given beauty & sexuality
Rebellion	Submission
And so on...	And so on...

To ***experience*** this power (God's good news for your intimacy and oneness), you both must:

Repent of (change your thinking about) the lies and false beliefs that have crept into your view of sexual intimacy. The problem is that most of us never really repent. We say we know God's plan is the best, but we keep our false thinking. The biggest challenge of this book is for husbands and wives to really exchange their thinking for the truth that God has a better idea for our intimacy.

Once you have "put off" false beliefs, you can then:

Believe (trust) that God created sexual intimacy as a tool for greater oneness and that with His help, you can take your romance and sex life to greater levels of oneness.

Once we believe the truth, how do we live it out? That's what the next chapter is about!

Chapter Six
A – Set an Action Plan
Commit to Hot Pursuit

Come, my lover, let us go to the countryside, let us spend the night in the villages. Let us go early to the vineyards to see if the vines have budded, if their blossoms have opened, and if the pomegranates are in bloom—there I will give you my love.
—The Greatest Song 7:11-12

...faith by itself, if it is not accompanied by action, is dead.
—James 2:17

And when I take your hand
I'll watch my heart set sail
I'll take my trembling fingers
And I'll lift up your veil
Then I'll take you home
And with wild abandon
Make love to you just like a true companion
You are my true companion
I got a true companion
True companion.
—Marc Cohn,
Lyrics to "True Companion"

Excerpted from a letter from David to Katie, Fall 2007

Repeatedly the New Testament urges, Repent/Believe/Walk. For me, walking in God's truth means I need to commit to lead us to greater intimacy. I sometimes get shy again because I base my confidence on your response instead of trusting that I am called to be the leader and that you will follow where I lead us even if it seems like unfamiliar ground to you at first. For you, walking in God's truth is believing you are a beautiful daughter of God who is absolutely desirable to me.

We've already been making great progress in experiencing the gospel, and I want to say again that I am so thankful for a godly wife who loves the Lord and submits to Him. I want to encourage us that part of my role as the leader is to keep making our marriage the best it can be...not taking for granted where we are, but also never settling in light of where we could be.

> ## A Wife's Take
> I treasure these words from Dave. They have the ring of truth. And I know they come from a heart that purely wants both of us to experience the holiness and depth of joy that marriage is meant to be.
>
> Dave has been leading me out of my comfort zone for fifteen years, and without a doubt, we are—and I am—better for it. My prayer this chapter is for wives to trust their husbands (and ultimately God).
>
> My prayer for husbands is for you to walk worthy of your high calling as a husband, thereby earning your wife's trust—and that by trusting God and each other, you would both take bold and godly action for the good of your marriage.

Up to this point, you've laid a relational (*Learn About Your Mate*) and spiritual (*Experience the Gospel*) foundation for a whole new way of doing intimacy, one based on the needs of your spouse and truth of God's Word instead of insecurity/selfishness and the lies of the enemy. But for you to experience this new God-intended soul intimacy, you actually have to *do* something. After

Scripture tells us to repent and believe, it emphasizes the necessity to walk in (live out) this new life.[132]

The power of the *Set an Action Plan* stage of the LEAD process lies in both of you agreeing to a specific, concrete plan of action. You've gained new life-changing insight from each other by talking openly about intimate things you've likely never shared before. And then, you've experienced the gospel—changing your thinking and reaffirming your belief in God's design for sex.

You're now ready to commit to make some changes together in courting and lovemaking!

A Warning

Let me issue a strong warning here: do not blow all your progress so far by failing to turn it into real action in your marriage. In this hard-to-talk-about area, major breakthroughs and headway are lost when you get to a new level of understanding but then fail to turn it into actual progress.

If you don't use it, you'll lose it. There's a clear spiritual reason why this is true. Jesus explained it to his disciples in the Parable of the Soils.

In Matthew 13, Jesus tells the parable of a sower spreading seed to yield a harvest. The variable that affects the crop yield is the condition of the soil that receives the seed. Three types of soil, Jesus says, are poor soil—but the final dirt, the "good soil," bears fruit from the "word of the Kingdom" (the gospel) that has been sown into it.

How does this apply to God's good news for your intimacy in marriage? The "word of the Kingdom" concerning intimacy has been planted in your hearts through what we've learned so far.

---

[132] Ephesians 4:1, Colossians 1:10, and 1 Thessalonians 2:12 among many others.

The great question now is, *What kind of soil will you, husband and wife, be?* Consider Matthew 13:19:

> *"When anyone hears the word of the kingdom and does not* **understand** *it, the evil one comes and snatches away what has been sown in his heart. This is the one on whom seed was sown beside the road."*

Jesus says the one who does not *understand* the truth will have what has been sown in his or her heart snatched away by the Evil One, just like a bird grabs a seed before it can be implanted in the ground. The Greek word *suniemi* ("understand" in this verse) means literally to "bring together" or to gain insight into something. The Bible often points out the importance of understanding/gaining insight/comprehending the truth God has to offer us.[133] Jesus' point is that you must incorporate new truth into your life ("bring it together") in order for it to have any value for you. The alternative, Jesus says, is that our enemy will steal it from us. This is true for all spiritual truth, and we have already made the case that the enemy robs couples of the truth about the oneness God meant for marriages to enjoy.

Jesus goes on to warn that another poor soil is one who receives the word with joy,

> *But since he has no root, he lasts only a short time. When trouble or persecution comes because of the word, he quickly falls away.*[134]

This soil represents a hearer who lets the pressures of the world threaten the fragile new truth just received. Time pressures and competing interests in our society

---

[133] Isaiah 6, Matthew 13:14-17, Mark 8:17, Ephesians 5:17, among others.
[134] Matthew 13:21.

that would keep you from acting on newfound insight are two of the dangers you will face in implementing greater soul intimacy.

The third soil is a hearer who allows his or her own sinful flesh ("worry of the world and deceitfulness of wealth"[135]) to choke out truth, and it "becomes unfruitful." For the good news about intimacy, fleshly impediments can be insecurity, false beliefs, selfishness, or other "thorns" of the flesh.

But the point of the parable is this: *be good soil*. In your marriage, hear the Word, understand it (gain actionable insight from it), and you will bear abundant fruit in your relationship.

So, use it or lose it! Trust me, you will lose all enthusiasm for what God has already shown you if you don't follow through with an action plan. Our enemy will see to that by snatching away what you have learned.

> *The point of the parable is this: Be good soil!*

Chunk It All

Also, don't expect to go from your current level of intimacy to the ideal expression of oneness in one step. This is a lifelong process. The world, the flesh, and the Devil have been stealing intimacy from you your whole married life. You shouldn't expect to have more frequent, free, passionate, romantic, fun, experimental, and uninhibited sex by next Tuesday if you are starting from a lowest common denominator plateau today.

However, you *can* move to a better plateau on the way to ideal oneness by next month if you focus on a specific action plan to get you a few steps ahead instead of ten. And then there's the month after that.

---

[135] Matthew 13:22.

Remember how to eat an elephant? One bite at a time. Don't overestimate how much progress you can make in one month, but also don't underestimate how much progress you can make in six months of intentional bite-sized chunks of action. A good rule of thumb is to commit to only what you can implement in one month, or two months if you have kids.

How do you eat an elephant? One bite at a time.

Take what works well for you and increases true intimacy, and make that a habit; discard what doesn't. That's how you get from one plateau to another on your way to soul oneness.

Taking Action

Setting an "action plan" for your intimacy may sound corporate and sterile, but all I mean is that you need to set real goals and take concrete steps toward whatever it is that the two of you have agreed needs to change. This may simply mean that a husband needs to step it up in creating an environment for intimacy to flourish by planning a date night, getting a babysitter, and setting the tone for the evening. Or it may mean something else entirely—we'll look at lots of possibilities.

Believe it or not, there's a biblical basis for setting an action plan for intimacy. The Song of Solomon shows that intimacy is not left to chance by a couple who are passionate for each other. The princess says,

I belong to my lover, and his desire is for me.
Come, my lover, let us go to the countryside,
let us spend the night in the villages.
Let us go early to the vineyards to see if the vines
have budded, if their blossoms have opened,
and if the pomegranates are in bloom—

there I will give you my love.[136]

Do you get it? She says, "Solomon, I know you want me. Let's spend time together (read: get away, go to a bed-and-breakfast, and go antiquing, hiking, or shopping). And Solomon...I will make it worth your while." That's enough motivation for this husband. How about you?

Making a Plan

Here's the assignment: what are you going to start doing, stop doing, or do differently as a result of your learning about your mate, repenting of false beliefs, and believing the truth?[137]

Start with what you've already talked about in the L and E stages of LEAD. Make a list of the desires that either of you had that surfaced in your learning talk. Look over the statements you both indicated that you need to repent and believe. With this information firmly in mind, you are prepared to set an action plan.

As with all aspects of your marriage, the husband ought to take initiative in planning, and both partners need to participate wholeheartedly. Leading doesn't mean doing all the talking or coming up with all the ideas. It simply means taking responsibility for making sure you follow through with the process. Husband, do not give in to the tendency to abdicate leadership because it seems hard to move forward.

Use wisdom and input from your spouse to decide what to focus on for the next one to two months. And don't forget to create the right setting for the conversation and pray for God's presence and guidance as you plan.

---

[136] Song of Solomon 7:10-12.
[137] Make your intimacy plan part of your overall life and marriage goals. (We make these semi-annually and track our progress on a regular basis.)

One of you will likely have a shorter attention span or be less comfortable with this endeavor. Don't push beyond what your partner can give. On the other hand, whoever has less tolerance for planning intimacy, do give it your best effort. The bottom line: practice oneness as you set an action plan for greater intimacy.

> **The bottom line: Practice oneness as you plan for greater intimacy.**

Setting SMART Goals

Remember the best goals are smart goals. SMART stands for the five characteristics of well-designed goals.

• **Specific**: Your goals should be unambiguous. When your goals are specific, they communicate exactly what is expected, when, and how much.

• **Measurable**: Without measurable goals, there's no way to track your progress. Motivation suffers if you can't tell you're moving forward.

• **Attainable**: Intimacy goals should be baby steps that require some stretching.

• **Relevant**: Your purpose is to increase intimacy and oneness in your marriage. Every goal in your action plan must be related to that ultimate goal. If a sample goal below does not promote oneness in your marriage, do not adopt it.

• **Time-bound**: The best goals have a specific timeframe attached to them. Without a deadline, your goals become less urgent and lose out compared to everything else competing for your time. "Someday" can become "we never got around to it" before you know it. We recommended action plans that last for one to two months at a time so that you can make observable progress and decide the next step based on feedback from the last plan.[138]

Sample Action Plan

The best way to define an intimacy action plan is to show you a sample. You may want to write out a long-term dream plan to keep in front of you at each of your talks, but only focus on a few goals at a time as a subset of the larger plan. This sample plan is by no means meant to be dogmatic or exhaustive—depending on your particular needs and desires as a couple, you should adapt your plan and pace to fit you.

These goals are organized from "foundational" to "icing on the cake" following the soul sex pyramid introduced in Chapter Three and reproduced at the end of this chapter. Husband, don't neglect the foundation. Wife, don't neglect the icing. Treat each of the sample plan sections as a springboard for conversation. (The commentary after each section should help get discussion going.)

This *sample* Intimacy Action Plan covers many aspects you will focus on over time as you make progress in intimacy. This is not a list to work on all at once. As you repeat your next cycle of LEAD (see Chapter Seven), you will set a new action plan and may adopt more or different goals once you have achieved the foundational ones.

If a section represents where you are and what you agree you need to do, feel free to adopt it. Otherwise, come up with your own unique plan that propels you to greater soul intimacy. Here's the sample:

---

[138] Information on SMART Goals adapted from *Leadership for Saints*, Part 17: The Value of SMART Goals by Rodger Dean Duncan and Ed J. Pinegar.

Intimacy Action Plan

I. **Agape Commitment**
   1. Husband—affirm to your wife that you want to love and lead her like Christ loves and leads the church.
   2. Wife—affirm to your husband that you want to follow his leadership.
   3. Resolve together to "do nothing from selfishness" but with humility "regard one another as more important than yourself"; "do not merely look out for your own personal interests, but also for the interests of others."[139]

God is by nature a giver. It's been said we are most like Him when we give. Oneness is achieved when a husband and wife are both givers.

II. **Spiritual Growth / Education**
   1. Study Song of Solomon together.
     a. Read one chapter per night.
     b. Husband—read a commentary on SOS and discuss it with your wife.
     c. Listen to "Peasant Princess" message series over eleven weeks together.[140]
   2. Keep reading *Leading to the Bedroom*.[141]
   3. Schedule regular LEAD meetings for the next six months (every month or every other month).
   4. Ask God to speak to you concerning your next step in intimacy.
   5. Pray with your spouse at least twice a week.

---

[139] Philippians 2:3-4.
[140] I can't recommend this series highly enough. You can download all eleven messages free at marshillchurch.org.
[141] See other recommended books listed in *Resources* for future rounds of action plans.

LEADing to the bedroom is a spiritual growth process. Don't short-circuit it. God wants to change you and teach you both. True intimacy is the fruit of growing together.

III. Heal Wounds from Abuse or Past Traumatic Experiences
1. Talk intentionally and lovingly with your spouse.
2. Wife—meet with a godly older woman or a couple of peers with healthy attitudes toward sex to ask questions.
3. Husband—begin to meet with godly men with healthy attitudes toward sex.
4. Read *The Wounded Heart* by Dan Allender.
5. Consider marriage counseling with a pastor or professional marriage counselor.

There is a wide range of wounds that can rob a couple of healthy sexuality. Some are relatively simple distortions of truth, which can be gently corrected by a loving spouse. Others that have left deeper scars, require a qualified counselor to help the wounded person walk through the process of healing.

It is beyond our scope and qualifications to deal adequately with abuse, rape, and other traumatic wounds, but we can't say strongly enough: there is HOPE and there is no shame in getting help!

As a young man, I was very insecure, and it was causing problems in my relationships. I knew something was wrong, but I felt too ashamed to get help. I finally became so miserable that I went to see a Christian counselor—but I was so embarrassed about it that I refused to file it on insurance.

How crazy that was! Within about four sessions, I had a clear picture of what had caused my problem—growing up without my dad at home due to my parents' divorce.

Even better, I also had some spiritual and practical strategies to overcome it. I also gained much greater insight into who God made me to be.

Needless to say, my view of counseling completely changed. Around the same time, I broke my ankle. I felt no shame in going to a knowledgeable doctor and getting skilled medical treatment to make me whole and physically healthy again.

In fact, the only shame would be if I had *not* sought healing and let my ankle set naturally in a malformed way. To drag a lame foot around the rest of my life when help was available would not be good stewardship of my body.

> *The only shame would be in not seeking healing.*

What some of you have is an emotional or sexual "broken ankle." You might not know what to do about it, but there are qualified, skilled people who do. If you sense that past abuse is causing a problem in your intimacy, don't go through life without getting help! God has provided a way for you to experience a "full life"[142]—and it would be a real shame if you missed it.[143]

IV. Courting

1. Commit to a regular date night (see 52-5-2 plan below).
2. Become a gift-giver (flowers, jewelry, little surprises).
3. Call each other during the day.
4. Intentionally be more romantic throughout the week—not just in anticipation of lovemaking.

---

[142] John 10:10b.

[143] If sexual abuse is in your past, it has probably affected you more than you know. I recommend *The Wounded Heart* by Dan Allender as a starting point, but please don't dismiss counseling. It could be the best investment you'll ever make for your own soul and for your marriage.

5. Hug and kiss each other when you leave and arrive home.
6. Say "I love you" often.
7. Make regular time to talk about your day every day.
8. Ask your spouse, "What could we do that would warm up our relationship?"
9. Spend "shoulder-to-shoulder" time with each other, taking turns doing the favorite hobbies/activities of your mate.
10. Find a hobby you like to do together.

Aligned Heavenly Bodies

One wife said, "For that [something her husband wanted to try sexually] to happen, the stars have to be aligned." Husband, align the stars! Get a babysitter, go out to a nice dinner, engage your wife in conversation— whatever it takes. Aligning heavenly bodies (yours and your mate's) is not that hard to accomplish, and it starts with courting.

I recommend a plan of 52-5-2. This is fifty-two weekly date nights including five "super dates" and two getaways per year.

A weekly date night can be dinner and a movie out, a budget date of romantic dinner at home and a DVD, or even a Saturday morning breakfast alone to talk. It's important to be consistent. Do not let funds be an excuse. Even if you have small children at home and a tight budget, you can do it—you just have to be more creative. Put the kids to bed early and carve out some time for yourselves or ask another couple to trade babysitting with you.

A "super date" is an extra-special date. It's not as exciting (or costly) as a getaway (see below), but it's more special than a regular weekly date. Every other month, you should consider a trip to the nearest bigger city to see a show, go to the local aquarium, or tour a museum. Super dates get you out of the rat race of regular life and help you remember that you are both relational, fun-loving people apart from your responsibilities at work or at home with the kids.

A getaway is just what its name says. This can be a full-week vacation or just an overnight bed-and-breakfast trip. It really does help to get out of town. Katie and I can both let down from ministry much better at least 50 miles from home. Getaways slow the regular insane pace of life and make space and time for sensuality. Go with the expectation that this is a sex trip, plus anything else that you enjoy.

We do two getaways just for us every year: one in January to recover from Christmas and do our annual life goal planning and one in June for our anniversary and to assess how we're doing on our life goals.

You may be wondering if getting away without the kids is strategic. On a tight budget, shouldn't you be doing family vacations for the kids' sake? Each couple needs to decide what their values and needs are. We do make family time with the kids often, but the best gift I can give my children—for their security growing up and as a model for their future marriage—is to love their mother. I need to get away and nurture my relationship with Katie *so that* I can give my kids the great gifts of time with them and love for their mother the rest of the year.

The best gift I can give my children is to love their mother.

When I preach having a weekly date night and annual getaways, I often receive pushback from husbands asserting that they can't afford that much courting. But what if courting could meet your wife's emotional needs, which in turn might increase the frequency of your intimacy dramatically (say, from two to five times a week)? Did it suddenly just become more valuable to you?

Changing the Oil

Date nights are like changing your car's oil. It keeps things running smoothly. No guy ever says, "I can't afford to change my oil"—we know we can't afford not to! At this analogy, one wise guy piped up, "but you only have to change your oil every three months!" Yes, it's a big investment, but the bottom line is this: do you want a high-performing (well-oiled) marriage or one that is always on the verge of breakdown?

You see, you have to compare the cost of courtship to the cost of *not* courting. Look at courtship as an investment in your marriage, the most precious earthly asset you've been given by God, and one that needs regular maintaining.

> **You have to compare the cost of courting to the cost of _not_ courting.**

If money is the issue, get creative. Trade baby-sitting with another couple. Order one entrée to split instead of two meals at a restaurant. Rent or check out DVDs from the library instead of going to the movies. Rearrange your budget to make date nights a higher priority than other things on which you spend disposable income.

Ultimately, you and your spouse should determine together how valuable courting is to you. We spend a lot on travel and romance but have chosen to do less in areas like cable TV and expensive cars. In countless marriages, a scarcity of romantic courting is yielding a scarcity of sexual intimacy, which is a terrible loss. One husband in our church put it bluntly: "Date nights are cheaper than divorce."

V.   Increase Frequency of Sex from ____ to ____ times per week.
  1. Consider your optimal lovemaking times and commit to have sex on at least two of them per week (i.e., Monday and Friday).[144]
  2. Intentionally reduce activities and get enough rest on those days because you have an evening appointment.
     a. Wife—take a nap if needed so you are ready for the evening.
     b. Decide how many evenings it is healthy to be out of the home per week and stick to it (include kids' activities, church, socializing, work, etc.).
  3. Anticipate the above days throughout the week.
     a. Husband—take out trash, wash dishes, bring home a gift, call, etc.
     b. Husband—ask, "What can I do to help? What will make your life easier?"
     c. Wife—pamper yourself to help you prepare.
     d. Wife—be waiting at door, send a suggestive email, etc.
  4. Wife—plan to bless your husband with a wife-initiated, unexpected bonus encounter occasionally.
  5. Husband—plan to bless your wife with, "I'm fine if you'd like a break tonight" occasionally.[145]

---

[144] Get specific! The point is to set a frequency that's specific for you and meets your needs as a couple. Specificity is what makes it an action plan instead of a wish list. Insight for how to set your frequency goal follows.

[145] #4 and #5 should generally be exceptional. However, the plan is to help your marriage not hurt it. Do not continue blindly with a plan that is not helping you toward oneness. Discover the cause of a problem and address it before you continue with any action plan.

Create Some Space

This is where the rubber meets the road. For too many couples, sexual frequency is dangerously low—and oneness and protection from temptation are the common casualties. Fortunately, though, frequency is also one of the easiest places to make a dramatic turnaround by implementing a plan. You probably have different ideas about the ideal frequency, but the nature of oneness is to put the other's needs first (both of you are to do that).

Great sex happens in the margin of life—so have some (margin, that is!). Don't relegate intimacy to the bottom of your priority list...if there's time, if you're not too tired, and if you're both in the mood, then you'll come together sexually. That's what most couples do, and it reminds me of my favorite line from Dr. Phil: "How's that working for you?"

Most couples have certain times throughout the week that are more optimal for making love. To increase your intimacy frequency, be intentional and commit to some of these times. Set an initial mutual goal of one to three times per week (moving up from where you are now).[146] Schedule these encounters for specific days of the week (e.g., every Mon/Wed/Fri). Do that for a month or two and then add in another day.

Make sure you agree on your weekly frequency for this season and the specific days of the week. This agreement is not an absolute rule that can't be broken, but it should be changed only sparingly and with mutual consent and planning. Your goal is to ultimately work toward fully incorporating meeting the needs of each partner. Many husbands have never known complete sexual satisfaction (not craving more), but often they are

---

[146] We recommend three times per week as great starting goal for many couples. That may sound overwhelming to the partner who has the lower sex drive. Use prayer, selfless love, and wisdom to determine a goal together. Systematic increases over three months will get you to the same place.

only a few short encounters per week away from being satisfied. Frequency is important! Scheduling sex does not eliminate the need for the husband to pursue romance, but it does let him know that his efforts will be rewarded!

Scheduling intimacy might seem like it would take the passion out of it, but that's not true! There's a lot more passion in regularly coming together and knowing you'll be together than in continually experiencing the awkward ask (see below).

VI. Overcome the Awkward Ask.
1. Adopt an open door policy.
     a. Open Heart
     b. Open Body
2. Wife—become a "yes" girl.
     a. If he asks, my first answer is yes.
     b. If I can't say yes, my second answer is, "Will you ask me again later?" (expecting to respond positively when he asks later).
     c. If I can't say yes later that night, my third answer is, "Can I do something to give you release even though I don't feel like having sex tonight?"
     d. If I can't help my husband tonight, my fourth answer is, "Can I have a pass tonight, and I promise we'll be together tomorrow?" (And keep that promise!)
     e. After the fourth answer, you will bless your husband if you initiate the promised sex, surprise him with it early (e.g., before work), and/or really make it worth the wait.
3. Agree on acceptable ways to satisfy the higher drive partner when the partner with the lower sex drive is not as ready.
     a. Spouse provide manual release.
     b. Spouse provide a "quickie" that's "all for you."
4. Husband—be a *hero* to your "yes" girl.
     a. Thank God for a "yes" girl!

    b. Don't take advantage of her generosity by falling down on serving, courting and loving—try to outdo her generosity.

    c. Show her appreciation in ways she appreciates—make her glad to be a "yes" girl.

Overcome the Awkward Ask

Wives are to be pursued—Solomon makes that clear.[147] But a wife should also respond. One of the most common tricks of the enemy is poor communication between a husband and wife regarding the "ask."

Often, a couple's love life stalls by not getting past the "awkward ask." Frequent rejection conditions a husband to bring up sex and ask less often. This works directly against a wife's desire to be pursued—not to mention that it also weakens the wall of protection that sexual release with his wife provides for a husband.

Conversely, in 20% to 30% of marriages, it is the wife who has the higher desire for sex.[148] She can become discouraged if her husband isn't naturally ready for intimacy when she is. For both of these cases, it's important to discover a good solution for the awkward ask. Read on.

Open Door Policy

In Song of Solomon 5:2, Solomon comes knocking on his bride's bedroom door. He greets her with tender words, "Open to me, my sister[149], my darling, my dove, my flawless one." He has sex with her on his mind after a long day of work.

---

[147] Song of Solomon 4:1-15; 5:2.

[148] Douglas Rosenau, *A Celebration of Sex* (Nashville, TN: Thomas Nelson, 2002), 215.

[149] "Sister" here is just a term of endearment used in those days. The princess is not related to Solomon.

Unfortunately, she refuses to unlock the door. Solomon goes away disappointed, and she ends up regretting the loss of closeness she could have shared with him.[150]

What couples need is an open door policy toward each other. It's helpful to think of your accessibility to your mate as a scale from zero to ten (see Figure 13).[151] Zero, of course, is a locked door, when one partner refuses to give to his or her spouse sexually. One is "pity" sex, intimacy given simply to avoid a conflict. Two is "duty" sex, which ranks higher because it is done with a heart of meeting your mate's needs, though the giver is expecting no pleasure from it and is not really excited about it. It is sex done in simple obedience to 1 Corinthians 7:3: husband and wife should fulfill their marital duty to one another.

Figure 13.
Open Door Scale

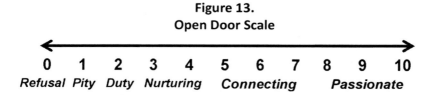

The door swings wider (three to four on the scale) with nurturing sex, sex where the partner has a warm heart to please and care for her partner with a higher need. He or she is participating primarily for his or her partner, but participation is "because I love you." Five to seven is connecting sex. This is where both partners are in it for the purpose of celebrating their oneness and to connect emotionally with each other. Eight to ten is passionate sex, those wonderful encounters where both partners are "all there."

---

[150] Song of Solomon 5:2-6:13 is a terrific love story of reconciliation after a disagreement over sex.
[151] This Open Door Scale is adapted from a continuum developed by Doug Rosenau in *A Celebration of Sex.*

A key concept to recognize is that the door can swing wider during the process as a couple "gets into it." Nurturing sex often becomes connecting sex as each partner gives to the other. This is possible because the door was open. So, in general, how open is the door between you and your spouse?

Having an open door is really made up of two factors, each of which may represent different struggles for each partner. Open door obviously refers to making your body available to your spouse. Is the door wide open, locked shut, or somewhere in between? Is an awkward ask required with the "Do Not Disturb" sign on the knob often? This is indicative of a closed door.

But giving your mate access to your body is not the only important aspect to having an open door policy. An open door is just as much an attitude of the heart as it is about an open body. Is your heart open to your partner? Do you share your thoughts, feelings and emotions with your mate? Does he or she feel your openness? Open your heart as well as your body.

I love the image of the open door. It represents close relationship. As a pastor, I have an open door policy with my staff and the congregation. I love to leave my door open. Anyone in the flock can come in when my door is open, share a story, get an encouraging word, and know they are loved. It's vital for your intimacy to adopt an open door policy (body and heart) with your mate.

As we've said before, there are issues that can make having an open door to your spouse a scary proposition. If you have been abused or wounded such that opening yourself up fully for your spouse is fearful or distasteful, then by all means, get help from a Christian marriage or sex therapist who is qualified to assist you in getting healing for such wounds. There ARE answers for sexual issues, and your relationship is too important to neglect the healing that can be yours. In this case, open your heart to your spouse and ask for his or help to get the healing you need.

Your relationship is too important to neglect the healing that can be yours.

Now, let's get specific about what an open door policy looks like in a healthy couple that just need a new perspective. Having a plan to overcome the "awkward ask" is one of the most successful things you can do for your intimacy. Often, the problem is a result of poor timing. A husband who hasn't been particularly helpful or appreciative (but has been thinking about sex all day) will spring a surprise request on a tired wife who has NOT been thinking about sex at all. If a "no" doesn't seem to have great consequences in the marriage, this, she thinks, is the perfect time to use it.

In this case, both husband and wife go to sleep a little resentful for their own reasons. Both probably would have legitimate cases—if marriage were a strict 50/50 contract. Enemy who came to steal, one. Soul oneness, zero. But I will show you a more excellent way...

Getting to Yes

There are many healthier and oneness-building alternatives to "no." In fact, you really should remove "no" from your vocabulary. Remember, the Holy Spirit led Paul to write:

> *The husband should fulfill his marital duty to his wife, and likewise the wife to her husband. The wife's body does not belong to her alone but also to her husband. In the same way, the husband's body does not belong to him alone but also to his wife. **Do not deprive each other** except by mutual consent and for a time, so that you may devote yourselves to prayer. Then come*

together again so that Satan will not tempt you because of your lack of self-control.[152]

What if you chose to say "yes" as your normal answer? When you schedule your optimal times, you are choosing that those days will be "yes" days. Mark it on your calendar just like any other appointment you plan to keep (in code, of course). Wake up thinking about it. Don't overbook your day. Remind yourself and your spouse of the day and tell him or her you're looking forward to the evening. Husband, this is your chance to make the timing/scheduling work for you. Bring home a gift or flowers; surprise her by taking her out to eat or writing her a love note.

Wife, sometimes your husband will need sex beyond your scheduled days. He needs to be able to come to you for stress relief, comfort, pleasure, closeness, affection, and all the good things that sex with you provides him. You are the only person on earth who can legitimately meet your husband's specific needs. Did God really make your husband's sexual satisfaction dependent on your cooperation? Absolutely, and it's a beautiful system that builds oneness and true agape love when each partner puts the other first. Ladies, you bless your husband when he can ask for and receive sex. I love Pastor Mark Driscoll's line on this: "You're not that tired!"[153]

But maybe you are. Does giving up "no" sound revolutionary and scary? It doesn't need to. It's really just a different way of looking at the same situation. Every "no" is really just a "not now" because he asked at a bad time for you.

See, it's not so hard...we just moved from "no" to "not now." That's progress! You shifted the rejection from your

---

[152] 1 Corinthians 7:3-5.
[153] Driscoll. "The Peasant Princess: Let Him Kiss Me." September 21, 2008.

husband to his timing. But you can do even better than that.

Many a "no" really indicates, "My mind was not on sex at all. I'd need to switch gears to think about being intimate tonight." Instead of "no," say, "Will you ask me again later?" or "Give me half an hour." This does at least two things:

1) It gives you some time to warm up to the idea.

2) It makes your husband realize he probably hasn't been showing love and appreciation to you and gives him the opportunity to adjust his course.

Stormie O'Martian points out that women often warm up to sex as it gets going (not so often before).[154] It's okay not to feel ready, but when you choose to engage, you soon realize how good it is!

Husbands, ask early (dinnertime is good). You know you're already thinking about it—don't spring it on her as you get in bed. (How's that been working for you?)

The response, "Will you ask me again later?" gives husbands a chance to set the mood for the second ask. Wife, when you use this reply, it should be with a pure heart of gearing up to be positively receptive when he asks later.

There are days when fatigue, emotions, menstrual cycle, etc. really make you want to "just say no." But you probably have in your mind an encounter with emotional ramp-up, foreplay, orgasm (and it takes me so long to get into it, you're thinking), cuddling, and clean-up—all of which may result in a short night's sleep.

Let me tell you what your husband probably hasn't. (In fact, here's a heads-up: for the rest of this chapter, I may push you and your mate's comfort zone by talking about some specific things you may not usually be willing to talk about.) When he asks for sex, often he just needs a

---

[154] Stormie O'Martian, *The Power of a Praying Wife* (Eugene, OR: Harvest House Publishers, 1997), 62-65.

nurturing release and a tender heart from you. If you were to say, "Honey, I don't feel up to anything big for me, but could I just give you a quick release?" he may say, "Who are you, and what have you done with my wife?"

If you were to lubricate his penis and manually stimulate him laying beside you in bed until he ejaculates into a towel, he would NOT count that as a "no." Total time invested by you: five minutes. Feeling of closeness from a husband who needed a physiological release and knows his wife cared enough about him to give it: priceless.

Often, he just needs a quick sexual release and a tender heart from you.

Oral sex or a quickie that's "just for him" are also ways to bless your husband on a night when you aren't up to more. A curt "no" shuts conversation and oneness down, while a short negotiation can often satisfy for today and increases oneness.

Very occasionally, when you're not feeling well, the kids have driven you crazy, or you're dealing with a heavy life load, you really won't have the emotional energy to give anything.[155] And with true oneness, a husband should want to honor that. Let's still not make that a "no"—instead how about "Can I have a pass tonight and let's be together tomorrow?" (Setting a specific time is good.) Keep that promise, and make it worth the wait.

Finally, while we're on the subject, you would make your husband's day (or month) if you were to passionately initiate with him on a day you're not scheduled or he hasn't asked. That's being a "yes" girl![156]

---

[155] If this is happening too often, you should evaluate your lifestyle together and make some simplifying changes.

[156] Some wives have been taught that the husband should always initiate. The husband is definitely the leader, but in the Song of Solomon, the princess often initiates also (see Song 1:1-4).

Be a Hero

Becoming a "yes" girl or "yes" guy is about giving your mate access to your body. Often, opening your *heart* to your partner is the key that unlocks the door and swings it wide. Webster defines a hero as a man of distinguished courage or ability, admired for his brave deeds or noble qualities. Your spouse needs you to be a hero (or heroine). A hero is the guy who anticipates and acts on his wife's desires for connecting, rest, and romance. He takes out the trash, puts the kids to bed, and meets her needs for conversation, acceptance, and appreciation. His open heart makes it easy for his wife to be an open door. When you're the hero, you're asking without asking. Communicating your desire for her in the context of meeting her needs should make your wife feel loved instead of used. A hero is not selfish. He is genuinely working to please his wife.

Husband, if your wife decides to be a "yes" girl, thank God! You are experiencing an important part of the "full life" Jesus came to give us! Don't take advantage of her generosity and growth by slacking in your pursuit. Instead, fan these sparks of growth into a blazing, passionate fire. Serve her, court her, love her—try to outdo her generosity to you by appreciating her in the ways she values.

In summary, a hero makes his wife glad she's a "yes" girl. This is what God had in mind—two people putting each other's needs above their own, and in this way, both partners are blessed. If she makes "yes" a lifestyle, you will be the most blessed husband in the world. Make her the most blessed wife.[157]

---

[157] For the 20% to 30% where the wife is the higher desire person, "Getting to Yes" can equally apply to the other spouse. If your man commits to be a "yes guy," thank God for him and make Him the most blessed husband. You be his heroine.

True Love

What we're really talking about with the open door (body and heart) is *agape* love—selfless sacrifice of oneself for the highest good of another. This applies to both partners. However, don't use these suggestions as weapons to get what you want or withhold what you have to give—that would violate God's entire intention for marital intimacy: to bring you closer together. Consider these two passages regarding *agape* love and let them really sink in:

> *Love is patient, love is kind. It does not envy, it does not boast, it is not proud.*
> *It is not rude,* **it is not self-seeking,** *it is not easily angered, it keeps no record of wrongs. Love does not delight in evil but rejoices with the truth.*
> *It always protects, always trusts, always hopes, always perseveres. Love never fails.*[158]
>
> *Greater love has no one than this, that he lay down his life for his friends.*[159]

Jesus spoke this latter profound statement in John 15:13 primarily about Himself and His willingness to die for His disciples (and for our sin). For a moment, think of His statement differently. Who is your best friend? Your mate, right. In the context of sexual intimacy, "laying down your life" is adopting an open door policy with your best friend. There is no greater love.

---

[158] 1 Corinthians 13:4-8a.
[159] John 15:13.

A Wife's Take

Adopting an open door policy is a powerful concept. Giving freedom for your mate to access your heart and your body is the essence of what God intended when he said "the two will become one flesh." And that's precisely why it's sometimes the hardest thing to do. The world, the flesh, and the Devil conspire to close the door and steal oneness.

If there is resistance (from husband or wife) regarding maintaining an open door, let that be a warning to you that something is wrong. If there is some past sin, lies, or abuse that make opening your heart or your body to your spouse difficult, intentionally take the time and get the help to deal with it. We can't stress this highly enough.

Husbands, don't make the mistake of thinking that women are not sexual creatures...we are! We warm up slower, but we get just as hot. It's been said that there are no frigid wives, only clumsy, inept husbands. Being a hero is about taking the time and care to have us join you.

Most of all, this is a spiritual process. LEADing isn't about sex for sex's sake. It's about God's sanctification process in you—it's discipleship. You're both learning to "consider others better than your yourselves" (Philippians 2:3b). That's Christlikeness. Make it your goal to grow up as a godly husband or wife and not just selfishly get what you want. Use this whole process to learn to trust each other more than ever before.

In those moments when you find it hard to open the door because your desires aren't as high as your husband's, remember to ask the Holy Spirit for the guidance and strength to do His will. The Holy Spirit can resurrect your desire for your husband. Paul said, "And if the Spirit of him who raised Jesus from the dead is living in you, he who raised Christ from the dead will also give life to your mortal bodies through His Spirit who lives in you" (Romans 8:11).

Lower Desire Partner

What if one of you has a lower sex drive? Welcome to marriage! One of you will! (Typically the wife, but in 20% to 30% of marriages, it's the husband.) However, the very essence of *agape* love and biblical oneness is putting the needs of your spouse above your own, isn't it?

Perhaps the greatest "amen!" I have ever received during a sermon came in a marriage series when I humorously relayed that I'd found research that said that men needed sex every seventy-two hours. I think every man in the room cheered.

Shortly thereafter, a well-meaning nurse in our congregation told a group of ladies in her Bible study that what I had said was not true physiologically. Biologically speaking, I'm sure she was right—but she missed the point. The husbands in the room were literally crying out for their wives to understand that they desired sex more than they were getting it.

We know from 1 Corinthians 7 that sex in marriage is a protection from temptation.[160] I believe that one of the root causes of the pandemic of pornography in our society is the enemy taking advantage of men not getting enough sex from their wives.[161]

Countless married men are sex-starved and do not know that it is possible to actually be satisfied sexually. The enemy has certainly stolen God's intent for marriages. Increasing the frequency of sex—by creating space, overcoming the awkward ask, and saying yes—is one of the simplest—yet most powerful—ways to build oneness.

---

[160] See section on 1 Corinthians 7 in Chapter Two for details of the argument.
[161] I'm not letting men off the hook for sin but recognizing that a deadly trap has been set.

> **Passion Point…from a Wife's Point of View**
> Ladies, ask your husband if you've underestimated how often
> he needs/wants physical release. Then ask him how quickly
> you could satisfy him without even changing your routine.
> Blessing him in new ways will promote oneness!

We've talked some heavy stuff—now it's time to lighten up a bit!

VII. Make sex fun!
1. Lose your inhibitions.
2. Experiment with expectations.
   a. Try new things!
   b. Implement a weekly fantasy night.
   c. Teach each other.

Experimental Sex

If you've committed to increase your frequency, you're going to be having sex a lot more often. Why not make it even more fun?

Our great hope for your marriage is you are both realizing how you have failed at soul intimacy and that you are deciding that nothing will stand in the way of cultivating the oneness that God intends for you.

How do you know what is mutually pleasing to you both if you don't experiment? Many couples have made sex such a high-stakes game through scarcity that they don't want to risk trying something new this *Many couples have made sex a high-stakes game through scarcity.* encounter. Perhaps this describes you. You both secretly think that because this may be your only time together for the week, it had better satisfy both people—so let's play it safe and go with what we know. Come on, sex is a renewable resource. Experiment! You would have given anything to experiment without guilt when you were a teenager—now is the right time to do it!

Intentionally choosing to experiment with new things propels you to a whole new level of freedom in intimacy. Your newfound frequency relieves the pressure of both partners having to be fully satisfied every time—so you're free to experiment!

Even the sense of being adventurous and vulnerable enough with each other to try new things builds oneness whether or not any given experiment is successful in deepening soul intimacy.

If you have not experimented much in the past, there are sure to be new encounters that do promote feelings of closeness. Here are a few that often become taboos in couples' minds, if not in belief then at least in practice. As long as they promote oneness and do not cause shame, they are God-given gifts.

Quickies

The average husband needs sex more often than the average wife. The good news is that he can be satisfied in literally about five minutes. The stress release and warm feelings toward a wife that last long after a quickie are worth it. Five minutes! You're not that busy—and if you are, cut something else out. Bonus points if you do it before work. What a way to start the day!

Oral Sex / Manual Sex / Sex in Shower

These are things a husband may be craving and yet afraid to ask about because of past or potential rejection. It is not healthy to let these common fantasies be elusive.

Fantasy Night

You've heard of the "honey-do" list. You write down odd jobs that need to be done around the house so that when there's a free moment, your "honey" knows what to do.

Well, this is a much more fun version of that. You could call this a "honey-this-is-what-I'd-like-to-do" list. Here is a set of rules that work well, but feel free to establish your own:

1. The husband makes a list (though the wife is encouraged to submit anything she desires) to be cut up and put into an envelope or Ziploc bag.[162]
2. The wife gets to approve everything that goes in. (This is powerful; she's pre-approved anything that is in the bag! Oh boy!)
3. Draw one fantasy out on Monday if your fantasy night is on Friday,[163] so you both have all week to anticipate and prepare.
4. The wife gets up to three passes every week; in other words, when you draw, she can say, "I'm not ready for that this week," and you draw again. By the fourth draw, though, she will have picked something she is willing to try. (It helps to have a LOT of fantasies in the mix).
5. At any point, she can cancel if she decides this isn't the week for that (whatever "that" is).

Again, the purpose for this is for fun and to push the envelope a little bit for the partner who may be more shy—and to give the more adventurous partner a way to draw his mate along in a loving and playful manner. It is

---

[162] This makes your list easy to hide (from the kids) and portable when you go on trips.

[163] Our codeword for this is "Fun Friday."

not to be used as a means to force your spouse into anything.

What goes on the fantasy list? Great question!

Different Positions

If you're stuck in missionary-style-only lovemaking, you are missing out on the incredible variety God made it possible for human bodies to enjoy. Different positions create different sensations for husband and wife, and unashamedly trying them together for what fits you as a couple is an exercise in greater oneness in a class all by itself.[164]

Different Settings

If you only make love in the bedroom, you're missing the fun and erotic element of trying sex in different places. Try the kitchen table, the stairs, the bathroom counter, bathtub, the shower, the car, the backyard under the stars. You don't know yet if it will be great or not—but wouldn't it be fun to try without fear of rejection?

The things we leave unsaid to our spouse become more important than they really are. Ask your spouse if he or she has fantasies of making love in unusual places— then listen without judging. If the goal is oneness, and rotating around the house for variety would make him feel closer to you, wouldn't it be worth it to roam from the bedroom one night a week?

---

[164] For information on different sexual positions from a Christian source without immodest photos, I recommend christiannymphos.org, a blog by several Christian wives promoting marital intimacy. Search on positions.

Other Items for the Fantasy List

Wearing new lingerie, trying new experiences or activities, romantic ideas, fun dates, sexy ways to make love, being more vocal/passionate/visual when making love—your imagination is the limit to what you and your lover can add to your fantasy list.[165] The only guideline is that it should promote oneness between you.[166]

VIII. Make sex passionate!
1. Be "all there" when you make love.
2. Flirt with each other.
3. Teach each other what you like.

"All There" Passion

In the movies, sex is portrayed as an all-encompassing, overwhelming experience where two people are ecstatically engaged in each other to the point of losing themselves in passion.

A few years of marriage seems to tame sex, but it does not have to be that way. Are you missing some of the passion that you could have?

At the risk of oversimplifying, passion is the fruit of being completely "there" for each other, not only physically in the bedroom, but relationally there in courting and daily tasks, emotionally there to give to your spouse, sensually there to heighten the experience—all there. You've had moments when you know what that is like, and you've had moments when—not so much.

The enemy works overtime to steal this "all there" passion out of our lives (remember, he came to steal, kill, and destroy) by making us take for granted the incredible

---

[165] Get a downloadable sample fantasy list at leadingtothebedroom.com.
[166] We've already determined that anything that hurts, demeans, or shames either partner is the antithesis of oneness and is to be avoided.

gift we have in each other and instead focus only on ourselves.

The Importance of Flirting

Here is one way he does this: A husband plans to flirt with his wife and be passionate. He compliments the way she looks, holds her and kisses her. But he feels a little bit of resistance, so he tones it down. She responded this way because she felt a little self-conscious even though she really craves that kind of attention. Her insecurity makes her not "all there" in the moment. This response pushes him away, discouraging him from being "all there" for her again, because he felt rejected.

Unfortunately, instead of heating up all the way to the bedroom, there's often an ongoing series of cool-offs during non-sexual times. Couples miss out on cultivating greater sexual passion by unintentionally pouring cold water on the starting fire because of shyness.

The antidote? Value flirting and everyday opportunities to be sensual as catalysts to greater passion during sex. Be all there. Send flirtatious emails or texts to your mate during the day. Dress up for that date night. Look in each other's eyes. Be intentionally romantic during dinner. Turn taking clothes off and kissing into sensual foreplay. Heat up, don't cool down after a date.

Teach Each Other

Push through shyness and teach each other what pleases you. By all means, communicate it when your partner does something you like. Sex is not something you know how to do well naturally; you learn it together with your spouse. God designed it that way.

Summary

Setting a one- to two-month intimacy action plan is the key to moving from your current plateau of intimacy to the next on your way to experiencing the greatest level of intimacy that God has provided for a married couple. Base your plan on where you and your spouse are, and tailor it to where you want to go. Using specific action-oriented goals, move from a foundation of *agape* love to the "icing on the cake." Use the Soul Sex Pyramid (see Figure 14) to give you and your mate categories to set your own action plan. Once you've got a plan for the next couple of months, you're ready to move to the next chapter. It's a fun one.

Figure 14.
Pyramid Model for Increasing Intimacy

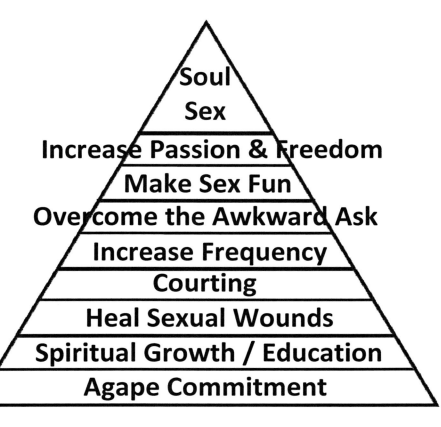

Chapter Seven
D – Do It and Repeat
Follow-Through & Continuous Progress

Catch for us the foxes, the little foxes that ruin the vineyards, our vineyards that are in bloom.

—The Greatest Song 2:15

Two are better than one because they have a good return for their labor.

—Ecclesiastes 4:9

Success is 1% inspiration and 99% perspiration.

—Thomas Edison

In his incredible business book, *Good to Great*, Jim Collins powerfully uses the image of a flywheel to capture the buildup and breakthrough process necessary to achieve lasting momentum. He says:

> Picture a huge, heavy flywheel—a massive metal disk mounted horizontally on an axle, about 30 feet in diameter, 2 feet thick, and weighing 5,000 pounds. Now imagine that your task is to get the flywheel rotating on the axle as fast and as long as possible.
>
> Pushing with great effort, you get the flywheel to inch forward, moving almost imperceptibly at first. You keep pushing and, after two or three hours of persistent effort, you get the flywheel to complete one entire turn.
>
> You keep pushing, and the flywheel begins to move a bit faster, and with continued great effort, you move it around a second rotation. You keep pushing in a consistent

direction. Three turns...four...five...six...the flywheel builds up speed...seven...eight...you keep pushing...nine...ten...it builds momentum...eleven...twelve...moving faster with each turn...twenty...thirty...fifty...a hundred.

Then at some point—breakthrough! The momentum of the thing kicks in your favor, hurling the flywheel forward, turn after turn...whoosh!...its own heavy weight working for you. You're pushing no harder than during the first rotation, but the flywheel goes faster and faster. Each turn of the flywheel builds upon work done earlier, compounding your investment of effort. A thousand times faster, then ten thousand, then a hundred thousand. The huge heavy disk flies forward, with almost unstoppable momentum.

Now suppose someone came along and asked, "What was the one big push that caused this thing to go so fast?"

You wouldn't be able to answer; it's just a nonsensical question. Was it the first push? The second? The fifth? The hundredth? No! It was *all* of them added together in an overall accumulation of effort applied in a consistent direction. Some pushes may have been bigger than others, but any single heave—no matter how large—reflects a small fraction of the entire cumulative effect upon the flywheel.[167]

Increasing oneness in marriage follows the flywheel effect. Every little push toward greater soul intimacy—whether it be conversation, courting, or sexual encounters—builds up a stronger oneness. In fact, it's not so much the intensity of a single encounter that brings greater lasting oneness, but the buildup over time of pushing the wheel unceasingly in the same direction.

Said another way, marriage oneness is the warmth of a campfire, carefully arranged to take advantage of fuel, oxygen, and heat from embers. With everything working together toward creating heat, the fire burns hotter and hotter.

With everything working toward creating heat, the fire burns hotter and hotter.

---

[167] Jim Collins, *Good to Great* (New York: HarperCollins Publishers, 2001), 164-5.

Work on your Marriage

Church planters like myself everywhere have taken to heart some advice from another business book called *The E-Myth Revisited* by Michael Gerber. Gerber says to work on your business, not just in it.[168] In church planting, it means to prioritize working on the ministry system— policies, equipping of the saints, developing the staff, etc.—increasing the potential to do more and better ministry instead of simply continuing to do ministry at the current level of (in)efficiency. It means feeding the goose that lays the golden eggs instead of killing it.

The principle is just as important for your marriage: work on your marriage, not just in it. Amid all your errand-running, kid-rearing, and living-making, prioritize the union that makes everything else meaningful and possible.

After the first three steps of the LEAD process, you have all the pieces in place to increase sexual intimacy leading to oneness. But you have to actually *do* the plan, day in and day out, week in and week out, in order to have increased oneness as a result of your relational and spiritual insight and practical planning.

It Takes Discipline

Do It and Repeat boils down to discipline, committing to live out the intimacy action plan you agreed to—getting so serious about building soul oneness in your marriage that it becomes second nature.

It won't come easy. Our enemy fights hard with all the schemes we've examined previously to keep soul sex from becoming a habit in your marriage. The world, the flesh, and the Devil are all aligned to block your progress at every turn.

---

[168] Michael Gerber, *The E-Myth Revisited* (New York: HarperCollins Publishers, 1995), 98.

Thankfully, though, you don't have to muster up **self-discipline** to grow closer in your marriage. Discipline to grow in your marriage or mature in any area of life is actually a fruit of the Holy Spirit working in you. Galatians 5:22-23 says,

> But the fruit of the Spirit is love, joy, peace, patience, kindness, goodness, faithfulness, gentleness and **self-control**. Against such things there is no law.

So if you've tried and failed at being disciplined in developing intimacy, consider whether you've been trying with your own strength in the flesh. If so, declare your dependence on the Lord to make progress, and allow Him to "try" through you.[169] You'll find that He really is there to bring about all the fruit promised in this verse as soon as we rely on Him instead of trying in the flesh.

Breaking Through Plateaus

Thus far, we've outlined a relational (*Learn About Your Mate*), spiritual (*Experience the Gospel*), and action-oriented (*Set an Action Plan*) process for increasing intimacy the way God intended it in marriage. You've been encouraged to

- take an honest look at your current level of intimacy
- dream together about what could be (God's design)
- get on the same page
- experience God's good news for your marriage
- make a specific action plan to move you toward a greater level of intimacy.

---

[169] If you believe this is your particular area of struggle, work carefully through Chapter Five, *Experience the Gospel*, again and see the *Epilogue*.

Now is the time to do it—start pushing that flywheel! Where you are now in your sexual intimacy and oneness is a plateau that you have become stuck on. It may not feel like a plateau because you've been there for years. But I believe most marriages are one major adjustment from breaking through their current intimacy plateau to a greater level of intimacy. Men, you are called to lead your wives past your current plateau and get to the next level of intimacy and oneness. Ladies, you are called to follow your husband's leadership. This way, you don't get stuck on a lower plateau for the rest of your life.

> *Most marriages are one major adjustment away from a greater level of intimacy.*

Figure 15 depicts a typical series of plateaus a couple might experience while LEADing to greater oneness. This couple is starting at a potentially dangerous low frequency of two times per month. This starting plateau could be dramatically improved by implementing a one-to-two month action plan to get to Plateau #2, a much healthier eight times a month frequency.[170] Perhaps their mutually agreed-on next step (after going through the LEAD steps) would be to move to a third plateau of committing to a weekly date night and the wife becoming a yes girl and the husband a hero.[171] One to two months later, (again after LEADing), they decide to experiment more intentionally with more erotic ways of making love, setting a specific action plan of things to try. This fourth plateau represents a huge advance in soul intimacy from their starting plateau. Incredible results for six months of intentionality!

The ultimate goal of each round of LEADing is to move from one plateau to another on the way to the

---

[170] Rule of thumb: give yourself two months to get to a new plateau if you have kids at home.

[171] See Chapter Six.

oneness God intended. What your specific LEAD steps are depend on your relationship, your starting point, and what constitutes oneness, soul sex, and met needs for you. For example, one husband may crave erotic experimentation more than another; another wife may desire more cherishing than another. There is no one-size-fits-all LEAD process.

Furthermore, this process does not exist in a vacuum. Life circumstances will come up that hinder progress. If you always have oneness as the goal of the process, you won't be frustrated when life throws a curve, but rather you can use that curve to show your spouse how much you care for him or her even if your best laid plans are going awry for the moment. Just beware that you don't let the busyness of life deter you from your path to greater oneness. Your partner's feelings are paramount, and true oneness will use Philippians 2:3-4 as a guide:

> *Do nothing out of selfish ambition or vain conceit, but in humility **consider others [your spouse] better than yourselves.** Each of you should look not only to your own interests, but **also to the interests of others.**[172]*

---

[172] All of Philippians 2 describes Christ's character and love. Christ-likeness in each partner leads to oneness.

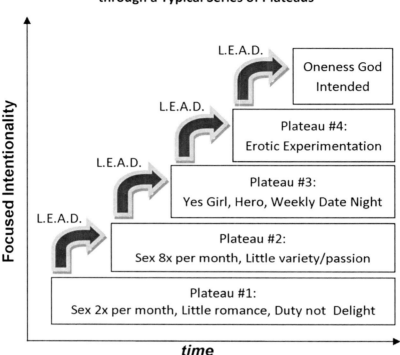

**Figure 15. The LEAD Process
through a Typical Series of Plateaus**

Make it Personal

Make a year-long, plateau-busting plan. Grow spiritually in the area of sex by studying resources in the Appendix. Work on frequency and dating. Men, work on expressing yourself verbally to your bride, and make deeper conversations a regular part of your week. Become a hero, serving your wife and a "yes" man to emotional closeness. Ladies, work your way to becoming a "yes" girl—and walls built up through infrequency and feelings of rejection by your husband will disappear. Work on intentionally having fun (variety of positions, locations, settings). Share your fantasies; buy some lingerie. Resolve to move toward complete soul oneness.

Do your one-to-two month intimacy action plan, LEAD into another plan, then LEAD again.

Why do we get stuck on plateaus?

The second law of thermodynamics has part of the answer. Stated in layman's terms, this physical law that applies to everything in the universe could be summed up:

Left to themselves, things get worse, not better.

Machines have to be intentionally designed and built; left alone, they rust and disintegrate. Dishes get dirty, they don't get clean. Houses get dusty, laundry piles up, air conditioners break, tires wear out...it's part of the original curse. Left to itself, everything deteriorates, nothing spontaneously gets more ordered or better on its own. Atrophy happens. It's part of the curse of the Fall.

So, just because you enthusiastically decide to LEAD to the bedroom one month doesn't mean that your spouse will remember and be absolutely on board with you the next. Life happens, atrophy happens, and you have to work to get keep from sliding backwards in your intimacy.

What to Do When You're Stuck

We've all been there. Despite all efforts to the contrary, there is a misunderstanding and things go wrong. When you have a miscommunication about intimacy, if you handle it wrong, you can hinder further progress because the hiccup can make both partners more timid about moving forward.

So what is the process when things go wrong?

It's still LEAD.

Here are L, E, A, and D restated with a specific emphasis on breaking through an impasse.

Step One. *Learn about your mate.* Focus on the fact that there has been a misunderstanding. What specifically has been misunderstood? Are there smokescreens that are clouding the real issue? Is it time to get away for a relaxing, romantic getaway to facilitate intimate communication? Make a commitment to lead through any misunderstanding.

Step Two. *Experience the gospel.* What false beliefs do you need to repent of? Don't try to be the Holy Spirit for your spouse, but definitely don't try to hide from His convicting work in your own life. Do you need to forgive your spouse for something or ask for forgiveness? What truth do you need to believe to break through your current plateau?

Step Three. *Set an Action plan.* Identify where you are on the soul sex pyramid and use the sample action plan in the last chapter to help you come up with practical action steps for your relationship that will propel you to greater intimacy.

Step Four. *Do it and repeat.* Commit to follow through with the relational, spiritual, and practical knowledge you have gained to move toward greater intimacy. By thinking through these steps just now, you and your partner should be able to put into words what obstacle is keeping you at your current plateau.

Passion Point

Writing a heart-felt bare-all letter is a great way to get out feelings that are hard to talk about in person. Instead of giving the letter to your mate to read, consider reading it aloud to him or her. You can explain something that is unclear, plus you have the benefit of tone of voice. This could be the key to getting unstuck.

Don't forget to Celebrate!

You can't work on everything at once. There is no reason to get frustrated as long as you're making progress. And don't forget to celebrate the progress you make. This is a fun, lifelong journey together, and it's really not so much about the destination as it is about the trip and getting there together. Rejoice that you are growing closer together and savor every intimate moment. Maybe you're not where you want to be yet, but thank God, you're not where you were!

A Wife's Take

It's important to view the *LEAD* process as a blueprint, not a strait jacket. Stress in your life often affects how you feel about intimacy—and unfortunately, life is full of stressful seasons. Grief over a loss, the arrival of a new baby, or any heavy life load can trigger a seasonal setback for one partner or the other. These times will make it harder to see the value and big picture of moving toward greater oneness in your emotional and physical intimacy. But the good news is that seasons change!

When hard times come, a spouse needs to have grace and understanding for the other who is cooling off; approach your partner gently and not demanding ("Love is patient; love is kind..."). Be part of his or her solution, not the problem—don't *increase* the stress!

I have more good news—it is much easier to recover from a seasonal setback after you have begun working through the LEAD process than before. Since you have already laid the foundation of communication and vulnerability, you won't lose all your progress. If one of you needs a break, then agree to take a month off from "doing" the plan and decide together that you will catch up next month! Think of it like a rest stop on the road trip to oneness.

Epilogue
The Greatest Challenge You'll Face—And How to Overcome It

The week I began preaching the Song of Solomon to my congregation, I heard about three pastors who fell morally. We are fallen creatures in a fallen world under attack by Satan—especially in the sexual arena.

For so many Christian couples, I grieve the loss of the great joy sex in marriage is supposed to be for a lifetime together. I grieve for the newly married couple who bring baggage with them. I grieve for the couple who've let the spark fade under the harsh wind of busyness. I grieve for the marriage on the brink of divorce, where soul sex long ago lost out to hurtful words and angry outbursts.

But even in my grief, I have great hope.

A Soul Sex Reformation

Martin Luther reclaimed the Grace Alone gospel by proclaiming a truth that had been obscured in his day. The result was no less than the turnaround of the church.

We again live in a day where God's gracious truth has been obscured by a culture blinded by God's enemy. It is our prayer that Christian couples will rediscover wonderful, passionate, soul-unifying sex that God intended and in doing so, we will see a reformation of marriage. If marriage was reformed among all Christians, and sex was restored to its proper place as a

God-given gift in marriage to be stewarded well, imagine what that would do for the church.

I have a dream that all our friends and family would come to us, as believers, for advice on marriage and sex. Wouldn't that be a great set of questions to get to answer? And wouldn't it lead to more questions about the wonderful God who made such a gift? This first depends on your marriage breaking through to soul sex. And that hinges on you overcoming your greatest challenge.

The Greatest Challenge You'll Face

I don't know what the greatest challenge is that you as an individual couple will face. It depends on your background, your temperament, your wounds, your starting point, the health of your relationship...and the list goes on.

However, I do know with certainty that there will be a "one thing" that tends to hold you back. Whatever it is, it's the enemy's grip on your marriage, holding you back from soul sex. It's the silence of Adam keeping you from leading to the bedroom. It's the shame of Eve resisting giving yourself fully to your husband.

So, what is your "one thing" that's holding you back? If you've just read through this book for the first time, and are just starting to LEAD, you may not know yet. But if you work together on the LEAD process, I promise you'll know in three months.

It may be busyness or an ongoing battle with shame. It could be that you'll have a hard time with discipline. The world may have convinced a wife of a lie about body image, or perhaps it will be harder to shake that male passivity than seems possible. Whatever it is, for you, it'll seem like a deal breaker, and you won't think you'll be able to experience soul sex the way God designed. You'll be tempted to conclude that the effects of the Fall were just too great.

And Then Comes Grace

After fifteen years of marriage, I've noticed that, at crucial times, there comes a mysterious God moment. When the moment before, things seem hopeless, and the moment after, there is great hope.

Ask for that moment. Wait for that moment. Believe that God will send that moment, just when you need it.

In the pursuit of soul sex, there will be times when you aren't understanding each other, or it seems you're at an impasse. If the problem is that your spouse has stalled—your husband wants the sex but doesn't want to court you, for instance—you take that request to God. Or if your wife just doesn't think she can overcome the shame her mind has associated with freer sex, don't pressure her (or go passive and sulk)—you ask God for His mysterious moment.

Maybe you've found yourself holding this book during a period when your marriage feels like it's about to completely crash, and frankly, having better sex seems trivial in light of your heart-rending situation. Beg God for His mysterious moment.

That moment is God's grace poured out on your marriage. He can do more in that moment than all the nagging or pouting in the world can accomplish. And He can certainly do more than giving up will accomplish.

Set your sails to cooperate with the wind of the Holy Spirit when He decides to blow—and He will lift you up.

This whole book, without God's grace mediated in moments when all hope seems lost, can't get you to greater oneness.

You see, the hope I have for Christian couples is the hope of the gospel—that Jesus Christ can redeem all that has gone wrong in the Fall, starting with our salvation, flowing out to our marriage, and ultimately recreating a

New Heaven and New Earth with no sin and no enemy. All we have to do is trust Him.

So, ask God for His grace, listen for His timing, and go back to your spouse for one more conversation. Push through the lies and know that God is in sovereign control. He's never broken His promise to be with you. Even during your hard times, "we know that God causes all things to work together for good to those who love God, to those who are called according to *His* purpose."[173]

Your or your spouse's "one thing" is nothing compared to God's mysterious moment—His grace to restore what the enemy has stolen. If God is for you, who can be against you?[174]

May the Lord richly bestow His grace—those mysterious moments—on your life and marriage as you seek to grow in oneness.

Love,

Dave & Katie

---

[173] Romans 8:28, NASB.
[174] Romans 8:31.

To Learn More

If *Leading to the Bedroom* has helped you in your journey to oneness, you'll also find our website helpful. There, you'll find:

- Free downloadable LEAD sheets
- FAQs since the book came out, and you can leave your own comments/questions
- Links to other resources
- Even more resources, coming soon!

To find out more, visit
www.leadingtothebedroom.com

Resources

Driscoll, Mark. *Lovemaking*. A frank sermon with excellent exposition on the book of Proverbs' contribution to love and sex. You can download this message for free at www.marshillchurch.org.

Driscoll, Mark. *The Peasant Princess*. Excellent next-generation exposition of the Song of Solomon. You can download the mp3s of this eleven-part series for free at www.marshillchurch.org.

Feldhaun, Shaunti and Jeff. *For Men Only: A Straightforward Guide to the Inner Lives of Women*. Sisters, Oregon: Multnomah Publishers, 2006. Great insight for men regarding how wives think.

Kendrick, Stephen, and Alex Kendrick. *The Love Dare*. Nashville, TN: B&H Publisher Group, 2008. A forty day exercise to demonstrate love to your spouse.

Leman, Kevin. *Sheet Music*. Carol Stream, IL: Tyndale House Publishers, 2003. Leman's skillful treatment of sex in marriage.

Nelson, Tommy. *Song of Solomon The Art of Attraction*. DVD Series. This chapter-by-chapter exposition is great for singles as well as couples. Tommy Nelson is a great communicator; I led a small group in our church using this study and it was very well received. I want my kids to watch this series when they reach dating age. Cost: $125.00. You can also hear Rev. Nelson preach an abbreviated version of the Song of Solomon for free at www.dentonbible.org .

Penner, Clifford and Joyce. *The Way to Love your Wife: Creating Greater Love and Passion in the Bedroom*. Carol Stream, IL: Tyndale House Publishers, 2007. Written to husbands by a godly sex therapist couple on "what women want."

Piper, John. *Sex and the Supremacy of Christ*. Wheaton, IL: Crossway Books, 2005. Compendium of articles on sex. Theological as well as practical.

Rosenau, Douglas. *A Celebration of Sex*. Nashville, TN: Thomas Nelson, Inc, 2002. The classic text on sex in marriage. Highly recommended. I give this book to premarital couples.

Weiss, Douglas. *Sex, Men & God*. Lake Mary, FL: Siloam, 2002. Eye-opening look at sexual issues for men.

Online Resources

Christian Nymphos. www.Christiannymphos.org. Site by Christian wives that encourages Christian wives in the area of sex.

Leading to the Bedroom. www.leadingtothebedroom.com. Get downloadable worksheets, free resources and leave comments on blog articles.

Marriage Partnership. www.marriagepartnership.com. The MP magazine is now defunct but their greatest articles live on at this subset of Christianity Today.com Excellent marriage and sex advice.

My Beloved's Garden Lingerie. www.mbglingerie.com. Christian-owned online site to buy lingerie. They don't display offensive photos or ship in offensive packaging.

Scripture Index

Subject Index

-I-

immorality, 47, 51, 52, 54, 55
intercourse, 32, 46, 54, 55
intimacy, *ii, iii, iv, v,* 3, 9, 13,
  16, 17, 19, 20-32, 37-43, 54,
  55, 57, 58, 59, 61-70, 72, 76,
  77, 80, 81, 83, 84, 85, 86, 88-
  96, 98, 99, 101, 102, 106-109,
  116, 117, 119, 123-29, 132,
  133, 136, 138-49, 151, 152,
  160-64, 170, 173, 174, 179,
  181-84, 187, 188
intimacy action plan, 80, 81,
  152, 153, 209
Israel, *i, iii, v,* 7

-J-

Jesus, *iii,* 14, 23, 24, 25, 27, 44,
  45, 72, 73, 74, 76, 92, 93,
  105, 117, 119, 120, 121, 123,
  127, 129, 131-133, 136, 137,
  139, 140, 142, 146, 147, 169,
  170, 192
jon boat, 24
junk, 122, 124

-K-

kids, *iii,* 26, 46, 62, 67, 83, 85,
  86, 97, 98, 100, 126, 149,
  156, 157, 159, 168, 169, 175,
  184, 195
knowledge, 34, 105

-L-

LCD, 8, 20, 21, 68, 69
LEAD process, 4, 61, 67, 72,
  76, 79-83, 86, 146, 182, 185,
  191

leader, *iv,* 23, 42, 58, 61, 73,
  74, 75, 76, 84, 92, 93, 126,
  130, 132, 136, 140, 145
leading, iv, 19, 24, 42, 60, 61,
  70, 73, 75, 83, 88, 90, 98,
  108, 126, 128, 136, 139, 140,
  182, 191
LEADing, *v,* 82, 85, 86, 99,
  119, 141, 184
Learn about Your Mate, 3,
  77, 88, 145, 183, 188
learning talk, 77, 85, 86, 89,
  91, 92, 94, 97, 98, 101, 102,
  109, 111, 114, 115, 124, 134,
  138, 150
libido, 37, *see also* sex drive
lies, 15
lovemaking, *v,* 85, 126, 128,
  146, 155, 159, 176
lowest common
  denominator, 20, 23, 24,
  68, 69, 70, 125, 148

-M-

margin, 160
marriage bed, 16, 50, 135
masturbation, 52, 55
misunderstood signals, 108,
  109, 116
mysterious moment, 192,
  193

-N-

naked, 3, 9, 10, 11, 18, 20, 38,
  63, 90, 95, 101, 120
neurochemistry, 55
newlyweds, *v*

Order Information

Leading to the Bedroom is available at amazon.com.

For multiple orders, feedback, or seminar information, contact the publisher directly at leadingtothebedroom.com

InnerMan Resources, Inc.
116 Mallard Ct
Carrollton, GA 30116

LaVergne, TN USA
25 August 2010
194450LV00005B/9/P